A RUNNER'S **WORLD**® Guide

RUN FOR ABS

The 6-Week Plan to TORCH FAT & SHRINK YOUR MIDDLE

By Rachel Cosgrove, CSCS and
Erin Palinski-Wade, RDN

© 2018 by Hearst Magazines, Inc.

Printed in China

Photographs by Mitch Mandel

Book design by Maureen Logan

ISBN 978-1-63565-345-8

8 10 9   paperback

HEARST

⏵ CONTENTS

5 CHAPTER 1
Ditch that Stubborn Belly Fat!

9 CHAPTER 2
Run Less, Lose More!

13 CHAPTER 3
The Big Fat Mistakes Most Runners Make

17 CHAPTER 4
Prioritize the 6 Belly Fat Fighters

21 CHAPTER 5
Fire Up Your Abspiration

25 CHAPTER 6
The Run for Abs Plan

61 CHAPTER 7
The Run for Abs Menus

78 CHAPTER 8
All Your Workouts in One Simple Chart

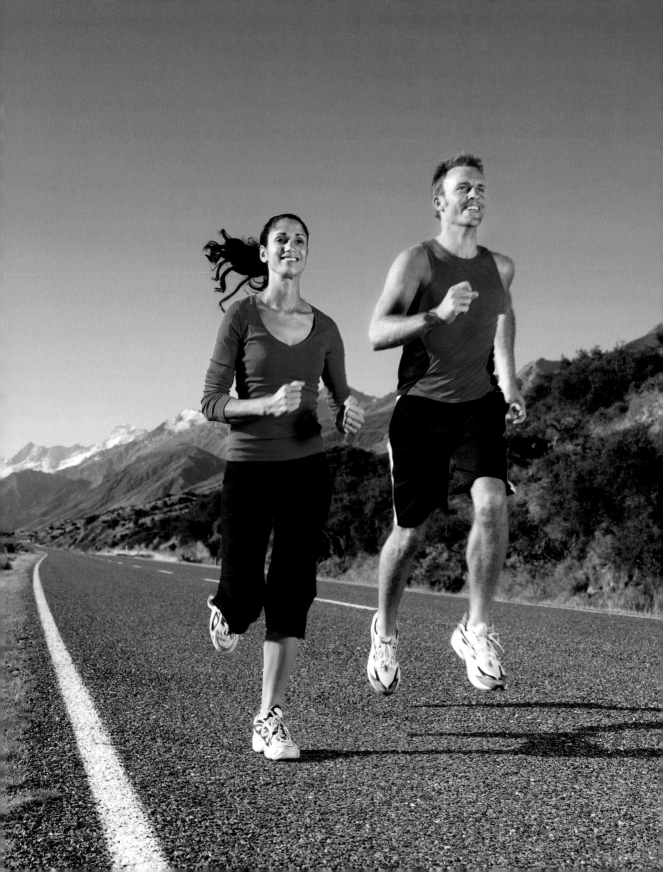

DITCH THAT STUBBORN BELLY FAT!

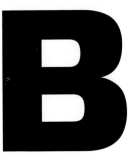**elly fat** is a lot like a bus station bathroom.

Think about it. What do you normally notice? In a bus station, it's probably the grime and the stench, not to mention the stray garbage that reveals way too much about the people who came and went before you. Chances are you don't think much about what you *can't* see: the much-more-dangerous microscopic *E. coli* bacteria that, no doubt, is lurking all over the bathroom door.

It's the same with belly fat. We obsess over what we can see and feel. We hate, for example, how it jiggles, gets in the way, and forces us to wear elastic.

In reality, however, the more invisible belly fat poses the true danger. This hidden fat can harm our health. It should truly motivate us to slim down.

The Anatomy of Ab Flab

Your abs are a sheet of muscles located in your abdomen. Along the front of your abdomen is the six-pack muscle, known as the rectus abdominus. It starts at the bottom of your sternum (breastbone) and goes all the way to the bottom of the pelvis. On the sides of your body, your external obliques create your waist. Also on your sides is the serratus, which connect your back muscles to your rib cage.

These are the ab muscles you can see – or, more accurately, *would* be able to see if it weren't for the ab flab that, no doubt, motivated you to *Run for Abs*. (A few other ab muscles exist deeper in the abdomen). The *Run for Abs* program will reveal those muscles by helping you to torch two kinds of belly fat: the fat you can see and the fat you didn't know existed.

1. **The fat you can see**. Called subcutaneous fat, this lard layer sits just beneath the skin. It's soft. It's roly poly. It jiggles, and it obstructs your six pack. For most people, this jiggly fat makes up 90 percent of the fat in their bodies, which is a *good* thing. Subcutaneous fat is relatively harmless. It even offers a few pluses. It keeps you warm in the winter, and it allows your belly to double as a pillow for pets and small children.

2. **The fat you didn't know existed.** This more sinister type of fat lurks deeper in your abdominal cavity. Tucked away underneath your ab muscles, visceral fat is easy to ignore. Unless there's enough of it to pooch your ab muscles outward, it's largely invisible. Solidly packed into the spaces between the liver, intestines, and other organs, visceral fat amounts to only 10 percent of the fat in your body. Metabolically active, it pumps out dangerous substances that trigger bodywide inflammation and raise risk for high blood pressure, diabetes, high blood cholesterol, stroke, heart disease, some cancers, dementia, even non-alcoholic fatty liver disease.

AB-VICE

A desk job will leave you with tight hip flexors and an unstable core. It can tighten your hamstrings, too, which flattens out the lumbar curve in the back, making it harder to absorb shock. The solution: take regular standing, walking and stretching breaks, and consider getting a standing desk.

For a variety of reasons, both types of belly fat tend to grow over time. After years of a desk job, muscles shrink, which slows metabolism. Hormone levels also shift with age, especially in women, causing visceral fat to grow. The good news: you can run away from both types of ab flab. *Run for Abs* will show you how.

The Right Way to Run for Abs

There's a lot to love about running. You've known how to put one foot in front of the other since age 2. You don't need a gym membership. The start up costs are low. And unlike many forms of exercise, you can vaporize hundreds of calories in a very short period of time.

But running doesn't automatically shrink belly fat. If it did, you wouldn't have bought this guide because your belly fat would be gone by now.

As it turns out, there's a *right* way to run off belly fat – and a *wrong* way. The right way includes a mix of workouts – hills, speed work, strength training. The wrong way includes just one workout: the same run you always do, at the same pace you always run, for the same amount of time you always run.

Do it the wrong way and you end up having to run longer and longer, only to hit a weight loss wall.

Do it the right way and you will:

Torch more belly fat. In a study published in the *Journal of Sports Medicine and Physical Fitness*, participants who did workouts similar to what's recommended in *Run for Abs* lost 3 times more belly fat than did exercisers who did their usual workouts.

This finding remains true even if you are carrying around a superbly stubborn form of age-related fat that many women refer to as "my menopot." Postmenopausal women who completed a program similar to *Run for Abs* torched more ab fat over 16 weeks than did women who exercised more moderately.

Keep off the fat. It's frustrating to gain and lose weight over and over again. Good thing fitness programs like *Run for Abs* have been shown to help you maintain your fat loss.

Get whole body strong. The *Run for Abs* workouts will strengthen more than just your abs. You'll firm your legs, arms and entire core, which will help to increase the stability of your hips, pelvis, and knees. This will help to relieve strain on your muscles.

Discover speed you didn't know you had. The mixture of speed work, hills and strength will give you more power in every step. Overall, you should be able to improve your running economy – the ability to use less oxygen at the same pace – by 3 to 4 percent, according to a review of studies published in the *Journal of Strength Conditioning*.

Prevent injuries. The *Run for Abs* strength training routine will help you to build a Kevlar core, which will help to stabilize your spine during running, preventing a range of injuries including knee problems, plantar fasciitis, low back pain, you name it.

Stay healthy. Workouts like the ones in *Run for Abs* have been shown to drop systolic blood pressure (the top number) by 6 points – after just one session – in people with elevated blood pressure. A single session can also drive down levels of inflammation and improve immunity.

Save time. We won't lie. The *Run for Abs* workouts are hard, but they're also incredibly

RUN THE RIGHT WAY AND YOU BURN MORE FAT IN LESS TIME, AND YOU HAVE MORE FUN DURING EVERY RUN. RUN THE WRONG WAY AND YOU'RE BORED, TIRED, AND FRUSTRATED.

efficient. You'll burn more fat in less time. The workouts range from 18 to 40 minutes – and that's including your five minute warmup and five minute cooldown.

Love every run even more. We often equate "easy" with "desirable," but the reverse is actually true. One of the top reasons we sometimes dread running has nothing to do with the effort and everything to do with boredom. Research published in PLoS ONE backs this up. Young men enjoyed higher intensity sessions more than moderate ones, despite the fact that they perceived the sessions to be much harder. That's because the constantly changing nature of the workouts helped to keep their minds engaged and alleviate boredom.

How to Run for Abs

As a runner, you're already well on your way to owning the abs you want. As we've mentioned, running is one of the best fat-burning activities around. But you need to run *the right way* to truly slim down and see your abs pop. Developed by coach and trainer Rachel Cosgrove, CSCS, and nutrition consultant Erin Palinski-Wade, RDN, *Run for Abs* helps you do just that. With this complete eating and fitness program, you'll:

Abridge Your Runs. To get abs, you need to forget about long runs. In fact, on this plan, you won't run longer than 3 miles at a time. Shocked? That's understandable. This is probably the most counterintuitive aspect of the plan, and we'll explain the reasoning and the science behind it in chapter 2. For now, trust us. You're going to pack a whole lot of burn into just a few miles.

Take More Days Off. You'll take three days completely off from running and all other forms of exercise each week. We can almost hear you yelling, "Say what!?!" Again, trust us. There's solid science to back this up. *Run for Abs* is incredibly intense, and this level of intensity requires more recovery. By taking three days off each week, you'll reduce your risk of injuries. You'll also go into each workout fresh so you can give it every ounce of perspiration.

Make Every Single Session Count. On this plan, you'll never lace up your shoes and plod around town on autopilot while your mind solves complex world problems, remembers what you need at the grocery store and has imaginary conversations with your mother. Instead, you'll squeeze the most out of every minute by cranking up the intensity. Each week includes killer hills and speed sessions, coupled with two total body strength sessions. If you are the kind of person who needs a little mindless running in your life, don't worry. You have the option of two short runs a week – but you'll do them after your strength sessions and not before.

Prioritize the 6 Fat Fighters. Research has uncovered six nutrients that can help you to burn belly fat. You'll learn all about them in chapter 4, and you can find dozens of breakfast, lunch, and dinner options that include them in chapter 7.

Now, we get it. A lot of this is counter intuitive, especially the idea of running less. That's why we've devoted an entire chapter to just that concept. Keep reading. We'll make you a believer.

CHAPTER 2

RUN LESS, LOSE MORE!

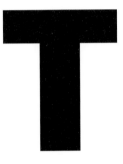 **There's a tired old** weight loss ditty that you've no doubt heard by now. It goes like this:

- A pound of fat stores about 3,500 calories.
- A mile of running burns about 100 calories.
- Therefore, you need to run 35 miles a week to lose one pound of fat a week.

For years, most of us have accepted this without question. In reality, however, weight loss is much more complex than that. After all, if things were this simple, all high mileage runners would have visible six packs.

So what's going on?

It all comes down to your comfort zone and the fact that nothing beneficial happens inside of it. If you tend to lace up your sneaks, head out the door, and hit cruise control, you're running in your comfort zone.

And we get it. It's blissful. It's easy. It's mindless. It allows you to fit in a run, take a quick shower and then continue to slay your to-do list – with no post-run fatigue to slow you down.

The comfort zone is everything many of us love about running.

WHEN YOU RUN LESS, YOU HAVE MORE TIME TO RECOVER. WHEN YOU HAVE MORE TIME TO RECOVER, YOU OPEN THE DOOR TO A LOT MORE INTENSITY, WHICH IS YOUR #1 SECRET WEAPON IN YOUR QUEST TO DITCH THE AB FLAB.

But it's also what has been stopping you from seeing your abs. Here's why. As your body adapts to running, it becomes a more efficient calorie burner. To get around this problem, you could just run longer, and longer, and longer, and even longer, all the while experiencing diminishing returns.

Or you could do something so counter intuitive that you won't, at first, believe it could ever work. You could run less.

The New Science for Torching Belly Fat

To shed ab flab, you must create what exercise scientists refer to as a "homeostatic disturbance." That's a fancy phrase for getting far outside of your comfort zone and into your high intensity zone.

Inside your high intensity zone, your heart pounds, your lungs suck air, and your muscles burn. You shouldn't be able to talk or sing. At this pace, all you should be able to do is continually will yourself to keep going. This is *not* your race pace. It's your "I can only do this until the clock tells me I'm allowed to stop" pace.

You do 30 seconds at this intensity. Then you slow down recover. You do another repeat. Then you recover. You go all out again. Then recover. When you're done, you're cooked, so much so that you need to take a day off from running in order to drain the post-run-fatigue out of your legs. *That's* high intensity.

And it's wickedly effective at vaporizing calories.

The caloric difference between a low and a high intensity session continues to add up long after your session ends, too. Exercise scientists call this EPOC (excess post oxygen consumption or oxygen debt), but regular folks have a simpler term: the afterburn. After a steady state smack-dab-in-the-middle-of-the-comfort-zone run, your afterburn is minimal. That's because your body returns to its resting state more quickly after a steady state run.

But when you crank up the effort, the afterburn lasts long after you've showered, dressed and gotten on with your day. The effect can go on for hours – even days – as your body struggles to resynthesize glycogen, restore blood oxygen levels, repair muscles, and rebuild protein. And it takes only a small amount of time in the intensity zone to turn up the burn long term. In one study published in the *Journal of Applied Research*, just four minutes of high intensity exercise (along with a 1 minute warmup and a 1 minute cooldown) kept metabolism up

AB-VICE

Forget everything you've heard about staying in the "fat burning zone." To finally shed fat, you need to enter the high intensity zone. That's 85 percent of your max heart rate. You're at 85 percent if you can only get out a few words at a time. If you can sing or talk easily, you're not pushing it enough.

for 24 hours! The study participants only burned 63 calories during the 6 minutes of actual exercise, but then they smoldered off an extra 297 calories from the afterburn. Put another way, they burned 5 times more calories as their afterburn than they did during the actual session! Even better: the afterburn primarily came from body fat.

In one study Australian researchers found that women who exercised intensely slimmed down faster than steady-paced exercisers who worked out twice as long. The women who did speed intervals lost up to 16 pounds, shrunk their bellies by 12 percent and their thighs by 15 percent, and gained, on average, 1½ pounds of metabolism-revving muscle in 4 months—all without dieting!

Intense running can also help you drop pounds by enabling you to eat less. Just 15 minutes of high intensity exercise has also been shown to reduce calorie intake, probably by dulling your appetite. Hard worked muscles release lactic acid, which is a source of energy, particularly for the brain. It tends to numb the desire to stuff your face.

By the way, high intensity running may also be better at reducing your risk for both heart disease and diabetes than steady state running. It's the clear way to go if belly fat is your #1 concern. We hope we've convinced you that comfort zone running is a big fat mistake. Keep reading to learn several additional mistakes that will hinder your efforts to see your abs.

ACCORDING TO SOME ESTIMATES, YOU CAN GET THE FAT-FIGHTING BENEFITS OF 45 MINUTES OF COMFORT ZONE RUNNING IN JUST 10 MINUTES OF HIGH-INTENSITY RUNNING, THANKS IN LARGE PART TO THE AFTERBURN EFFECT. THE AVERAGE PERSON COULD DROP ONE POUND EVERY 10 DAYS JUST BY THE AFTERBURN EFFECT ALONE.

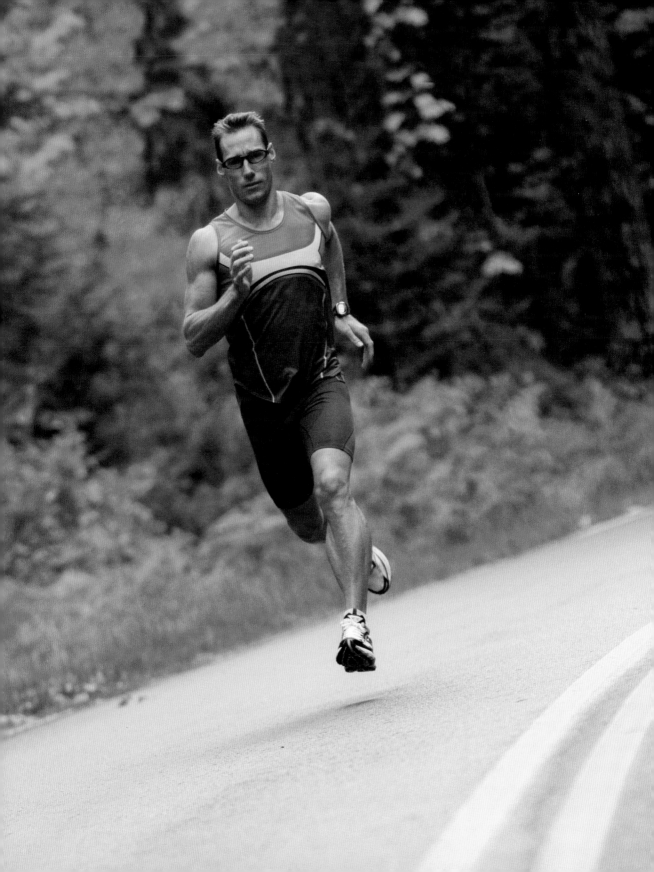

CHAPTER 3

THE BIG FAT MISTAKES MOST RUNNERS MAKE

We just told you about the dangers of comfort zone running, which is, by far, one of the biggest mistakes runners make when trying to shrink belly fat. That said, it's far from the only mistake. In this chapter, you'll discover seven more mistakes that may be stopping you from getting the abs you want.

MISTAKE: Running Before Strength Training

Many people like to get in their run before they strength train. That way they don't tire out their legs before the run. To ditch belly fat, however, you want to do the opposite. That's because you want to give your strength training session all you've got. This helps in two ways. One, strength training triggers an afterburn that lasts hours after the session is over. This afterburn is more effective if you push yourself to lift heavier rather than sticking to lighter weights that don't challenge you as much. Two, strength training builds stronger muscles. Muscle tissue is metabolically active. The more muscle tissue you have, the greater your calorie burn, even during sleep.

So lift first, run second. Give it your all during your strength training sessions. Then, if you've got anything left, go for a short, fast 1 to 3 mile run.

MISTAKE: Not Taking Rest Days

A day off from running makes a lot of us feel like underachievers, but rest is important. It's during rest that your muscles repair themselves and grow stronger so you can run and lift even harder during upcoming workouts. Rest also helps to repair your soft tissues. Cut it short and you risk an injury.

Too little rest also boosts your risk of having a slog. You know about slogs, right? They are those runs that feel unbearable from the first step to the last. Your legs feel like they're filled with lead. Your heart and lungs act as if they positively allergic to exercise. It may go without saying, but this is not how you want to feel when you're trying to crank up the intensity to 85 percent of your max heart rate.

On the *Run for Abs* plan, you'll take three days off each week so you can completely recover from your four high-intensity running and strength sessions. Don't do easy runs on your off days. Don't go for hikes on your off days. Don't cross train, either. These three off days will allow you to give each workout every ounce of perspiration. They're important. Don't skip them.

MISTAKE: Never Eating Fat

So, if you were around during the 80s and 90s, you've no doubt heard the old chestnut about fat having nine calories per gram, whereas carbohydrates and protein only having four calories per gram. While that's true, it doesn't tell the whole story.

You need at least some fat in your diet in order to keep your metabolism up. When dieters followed a low fat diet for four weeks, they burned 300 fewer daily calories than when they followed a moder moderate fat diet, according to a study in the *Journal of the American Medicine Association*. That's a considerable drop in metabolism. It's the equivalent suffering the consequences of eating an extra scoop of ice cream a day without actually getting to enjoy it. A metabolism that's burning 300 fewer calories a day is a metabolism that is standing between you and your flat abs.

Adding fat to your diet also can help to speed weight loss. People who consumed diets richest in olive oil, nuts, fish, avocado and other healthy fats lost more weight and had the slimmer waistlines than did people who consumed less fat, found a study from *Lancet Diabetes & Endocrinology*.

Welcome healthy fats from olives, nuts and seeds, whole eggs, avocado and fatty fish back onto your dinner plate. Use the mix and match menus in chapter 7 to guide your choices.

MISTAKE: Running to Eat

You run. You reward yourself with a burger and fries. It seems like the former should cancel out the latter, but the math just isn't on your side.

That's because some foods are loaded with more calories than most of us can run off. For example, the typical burger and fries tops more than 1000 calories. That's 10 miles of running, just to break even. Just one mixed umbrella drink can run you 500 calories. Are you really running five whole miles to offset each frozen margarita?

"Calories are the most important factor for weight loss," says Tara Gidus, R.D., a Florida-based sports dietitian and marathoner. "To lose weight, you need to take in fewer calories than you burn."

So flip the equation. Don't run to eat. Eat to run. Fuel yourself with healthy fats, lean protein, and other power nutrients known to improve muscle recovery, speed metabolism, and enable fat burning. And watch your portions. You want to trim about 10 to 15 percent of your calories to drop weight. The mix and match menus in chapter 7 will show you how.

MISTAKE: Not Sleeping Enough

Too little sleep muddles the frontal lobe of your brain, erodes your willpower, and sends hormones out of balance. Levels of the hunger hormone ghrelin go up while the fullness hormone leptin plummet. End result: you're hungrier, with intense cravings for sweets and junk, and it's nearly impossible to stop yourself from shoving food in your mouth. One study found that sleep-deprived people ate bigger portions. Another one found that they snacked more at night. Because levels of the stress hormone cortisol also spike when you are sleep deprived, the extra calories are likely to end up adding to your belly fat.

You need 7 to 9 hours of shut eye each night, especially when you're doing the kinds of workouts in the *Run for Abs* plan. Go to bed and get up at the same time every day – including on the weekends. And set yourself up for success by avoiding caffeine in the afternoon and blue screens (from cell phones, computers and tablets) in the hour or two before bed.

MISTAKE: Trying to Stay in the "Fat Burning Zone."

Perhaps we're starting to sound a wee bit repetitive, but this myth is so pervasive that it deserves a few mentions. Years ago, fitness experts told us that our fat burning zone was between 50 to 70 percent of max heart rate. It's true that, when we exercise at that intensity, our bodies mostly draw energy from fat. Because of this, it seems logical that we should make all runs slow and easy – or even just walk. But it's not that simple.

When you crank up the intensity, you burn less fat and more carbs, but you also burn more calories overall, particularly after your session is over. During the 24 to 48 hours after an intense session, the true magic happens. That's when fat burning takes over.

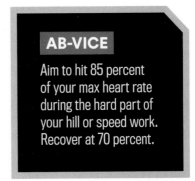

AB-VICE

Aim to hit 85 percent of your max heart rate during the hard part of your hill or speed work. Recover at 70 percent.

MISTAKE: Lifting Less to Get Toned.

Many runners skip heavy dumbbells in favor of lighter weights. But this is a waste of time.

To burn ab flab, you need a faster metabolism. To get it, you need to build muscle. To build muscle, you need to lift a weight that is heavier than your muscles feel comfortable lifting. It's that simple. When you go heavy, you create microscopic tears in your muscle tissue. Your body then comes to the rescue and fills those tears with protein, creating stronger muscles. Not only do stronger muscles make your body look firmer, they also boost your metabolism. Every pound of muscle burns roughly 15 calories a day, just to maintain itself. So lift a weight that's heavy enough that you struggle to squeeze out the last rep.

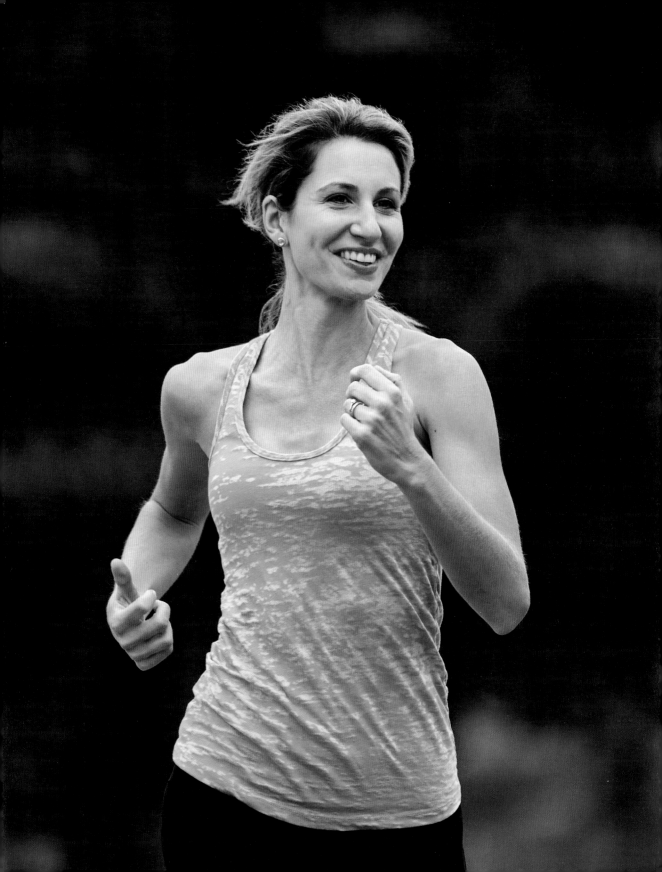

CHAPTER 4

PRIORITIZE THE 6 BELLY FAT FIGHTERS

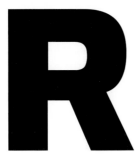**un for Abs** is about more than just running. To shed ab flab, you also need to pay attention to what you eat, too.

For one, as we mentioned earlier, it's all too easy to undo the benefits of a workout. Even if you slay 1000 calories during your workout, you can still manage to take in more calories than you burn. One large milkshake (packed with roughly 1000 calories) can erase most of your burn in a matter of minutes. So will the typical cheesy pasta dish at any number of your favorite chain restaurants. Portion control matters, no matter how much you run.

Two, certain nutrients work synergistically with your fitness plan to help speed your results. We call these the 6 Belly Fat Fighters, and we've worked them into your mix and match menus in chapter 7. They will fill you up, keep you satisfied, and help you to drop belly fat.

LEAN PROTEIN

Each of the *Run for Abs* meals are "macro" controlled to ensure you consume the right amounts of each of the three macronutrients (protein, carbohydrates and fat). Runners are used to hearing about carbs, which help to fuel your body and brain. In days of old, the advice for runners was to prioritize carbs above everything else. This is why pasta parties tend to precede most marathons.

Now, don't get us wrong. Carbs are important, but not at the expense of lean protein and healthy fats. You need a balance. In *Run for Abs*, we've provided that balance by ensuring that your macros for each meal align with these ranges:

30-to-55 percent carbs

20-to-35 percent protein

25-to-35 percent fat

These ranges allow you to get enough carbs to power your running, but also enough protein to fill you up on fewer calories. In one study, dieters who consumed 25 percent of their calories from protein reported greater between meal fullness and reduced late night cravings than did dieters who only consumed only 14 percent of their calories from protein. The increased protein percentage can help you to consume about 400 fewer calories a day without feeling hungry.

Protein may also help fight belly fat specifically by helping to keep blood sugar on an even keel. In one study women who consumed a diet with this percentage of protein lost more fat – including belly fat – than did women who ate much less protein.

RESISTANT STARCH

Resistant starch is a type of insoluble fiber that resists digestion. Your body can't absorb it, so it adds bulk and satisfaction to your meals without adding a significant number of calories.

Resistant starch contains 2 calories per gram, compared to the 4 calories per gram of protein or non-resistant-starch carbs. Put another way, 100 grams of pure resistant starch sets you back only 200 calories, whereas 100 grams of non-resistant-starch carbs set you back 400 calories. Those numbers can help you to see just some of the potential of this wonder nutrient. It literally allows you to slim down by eating more.

Rather than entering your bloodstream, most resistant starch travels to your large intestine where it triggers the release of fatty acids that help your body to burn fat. It also triggers the release of hormones that make you feel full. It's found in high carbohydrate foods like potatoes, grains and beans, particularly when those foods are cooled. Cooling triggers starch to absorb water and swell.

HIGH-SOLUBLE-FIBER FOODS

You just learned about resistant starch, which is a special type of insoluble fiber that does not mix with water and travels to the large intestine where, among other things, it bulks up your stool, making it easy to pass.

Soluble fiber is a different type of fiber that *does* mix with water to form a gel that slows digestion, making you feel full for longer after you eat. Like resistant starch, soluble fiber may also nourish beneficial bacteria in the gut, producing fatty acids that increase fat burning. In a 2011 study from Wake Forest University, people who increased their soluble fiber intake by 10 grams a day reduced belly fat accumulation by 3.7 percent over 5 years. In the mix and match menus, you'll find it in the form of legumes and beans.

SLIMMING FATS

There was a time, not all that long ago, when experts thought *all* fats were fattening. Now that thinking has dramatically changed.

Some types of fats – particularly the synthetic trans fats found in some processed and fried foods – are as dangerous and fattening as they always were. But other types of fat can actually help you drop belly fat, according to research.

The polyunsaturated fats in nuts, seeds and fish seem to be particularly powerful. We know this from a Uppsala University, where researchers asked young men and women to eat an extra 750 calories a day – all in the form of high fat muffins. Half of the group ate muffins made from palm oil (a saturated fat), whereas the other half consumed muffins made from sunflower oil (a polyunsaturated fat).

Now, everyone gained weight. That's no surprise, as everyone was overeating 750 calories a day. What's interesting is that the participants gained weight differently depending on which muffins they consumed. The men and women who ate the palm oil muffins gained mostly belly fat, whereas the sunflower muffin group primarily added lean muscle tissue.

In addition to the polyunsaturated fats in fish and nuts, the monounsaturated fats found in avocados can also help you burn belly fat. All of these foods are showcased in the mix and match meals in chapter 7.

FERMENTED FOODS

Fermented foods like yogurt and sauerkraut contain beneficial bacteria that's good for your gut. When you eat fermented foods regularly, you help to continually replace the supply of these beneficial bacteria, which can help to drive down inflammation throughout your body as well as allow hormones like insulin and leptin to work more effectively. In one study out of Japan, people who consumed fermented milk reduced belly fat by 8.5 percent.

ANTI-INFLAMMATORY TEA AND SPICES

A little inflammation every once in awhile is a good thing. The pain, swelling, heat, and redness helps your body to repair damage and fight off germs.

Chronic inflammation, however, is another story. When levels of inflammatory cytokines (a protein) remain elevated rather than dropping back to baseline levels, it interferes with insulin function, metabolism, and much more. That's why the *Run for Abs* mix and match meals showcase anti-inflammatory spices: cayenne, turmeric, and cinnamon. You'll also consume green tea to help keep inflammation in check. Green tea also contains antioxidants that may help to speed your recovery after a hard workout. People who drank 5 cups a day lost more belly fat than people who only exercised but didn't drink tea. Steep for at least three minutes for maximum benefit.

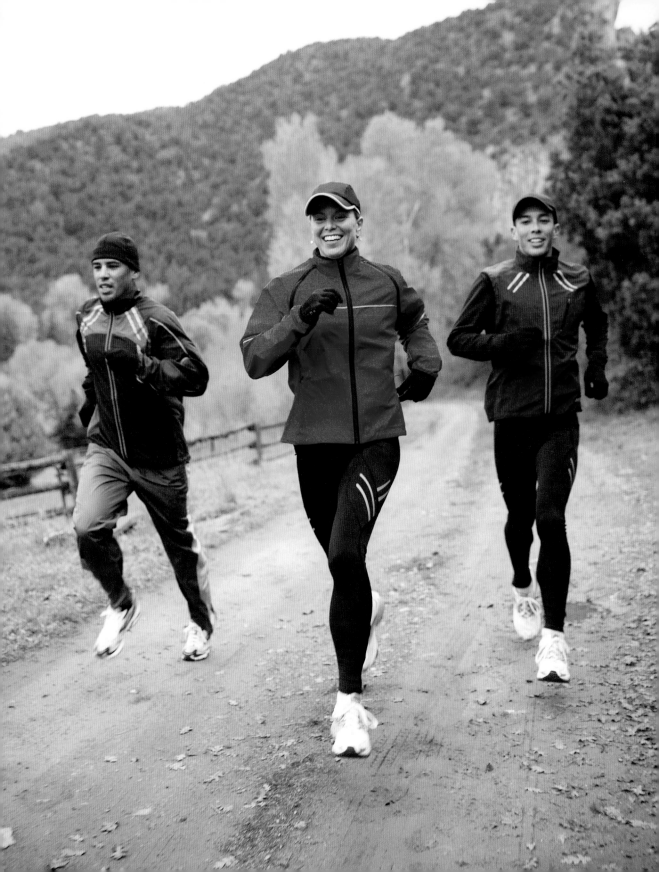

CHAPTER 5

FIRE UP YOUR ABSPIRATION

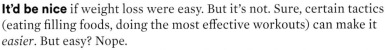

It'd be nice if weight loss were easy. But it's not. Sure, certain tactics (eating filling foods, doing the most effective workouts) can make it *easier*. But easy? Nope.

In reality, weight loss requires work: planning, shopping, measuring, chopping, sweating, grunting, and lying on your back with your feet up the wall as you pray that you'll feel recovered before your next speed or hill session.

It's hard, and deluding yourself into thinking otherwise will only set you up to fail.

Your success lies in anticipating and embracing the hard work ahead. It also rests on finding ways to continually remain focused and pumped – what we're calling "abspired." In this chapter, we've presented a handful of tricks from the field of behavioral economics to help you do just that.

Write Off the Weight. If you take a moment to flip through the *Run for Abs* plan, you'll notice that we've included space for you to write down what you eat as well as how your workouts went. If you're like many people, you'll be tempted to skip this record keeping. Don't. It's important, and incredibly effective. It can double your weight loss.

Overweight people who wrote down what they ate lost twice as much weight as people who did not do this record keeping, found a study done by Kaiser Permanente's Center for Health Research. That's because a food diary can help you become aware of everything you eat as well as help keep you accountable.

In addition to what you eat, you'll also want to write down your workouts. Keep tabs on your speed, number of repeats, reps, and weight lifted. Go over both your food and workout logs once a week to make sure you're staying on track.

Stop Making So Many Decisions. We don't make great decisions when we're tired, stressed or hungry. If you've ever devoured an entire bag of chips after the end of a long day, then you already know this. What you may not know, however, is this: we also make worse decisions after we've already made a string of decisions. Each decision wears us out a little bit. Eventually we become "decision fatigued." Once that happens, we tend to default either to impulsivity (*yum, that ice cream sure looks good! I'll have that now and work on shrinking my ab flab later*) or to doing nothing (*I'm too tired to pick out my workout clothes, so I'm just going to rest on the couch for a while*).

   You, of course, can't avoid all of your decisions, but you can avoid some of them simply by automating your choices. A few tricks:

AB-VICE

To pick up the pace, lean forward, pump your arms, and propel through your feet. Relax your arms, shoulders, and face, too.

- Plan all of your meals at the beginning of the week. It's easier for us to want the best for ourselves in the future, but harder in the here and now, finds research from Harvard Business School and the Analyst Institute. Planning meals ahead of time helps you stay future focused. It also prevents you from having to decide what to eat each evening while you are famished, tired and stressed.

- Pick a few *Run for Abs* meals you love and make them over and over. It's really a-okay to eat the same thing for breakfast and lunch every day, and it's also okay to make the same 3 or 4 dinners each week. This allows you to shift to autopilot both during shopping and during meal prep, saving your precious decision-making powers for when you truly need them.

- Automate routine tasks like getting dressed. You could, for example, follow Facebook CEO Mark Zuckerberg's example and wear jeans and a gray T-shirt every single day. Or, you could arrange your closet to make it easy to just reach in and pull out a complete outfit — no thought required.

Workout in the Morning. This relates to decision fatigue (see previous tip), but it's so important that we gave it it's own heading. In the morning, you're fresh, which makes you more likely to push yourself through those final two repeats instead of calling it quits. Get in the habit each night of setting yourself up for success for the following morning. Have your exercise clothes laid out and ready. One better: meet someone for your run. That will make it harder to turn off the alarm, roll over, and fall back to sleep.

Turn Run for Abs into a Competition. Consider what might happen if you signed up for and ran a Spartan or Tough Mudder alone rather than with a team. Do you think you'd follow through? Or would you wilt once the going got tough? Being part of a team helps us to dig way down and give every ounce to the cause. Perhaps you and four other people form one team, and you compete against another to see which team gets six packs the fastest.

Give Away Money. Many people set up incentives for reaching a goal. Drop 5 pounds and get a massage, that sort of thing. But what's actually more effective than incentives, according to behavioral economics, is the fear of loss.

In a study from the University of Pennsylvania, participants were asked to complete 7,000 daily steps. Some of the participants received $1.40 each day they met their goal. Others lost $1.40 each time they fell short. Still others were placed into a lottery that made them eligible to win either $5 or $50 a day and a final group got no incentive. The participants who lost money whenever they fell short ended up walking the most.

You can test this out on yourself. Consider this: Would you be more likely to successfully complete this program if you knew you'd win a free car by doing so? Or, would you be more likely to finish if you knew you'd lose the car you are currently driving if you failed?

Let a friend in on what you are doing. For every workout you skip or cut short, you have to pay the friend at least a $1, $5, $10 or more dollars.

Wear a Backpack During Your Craving Window. If you have a time of day when you just can't keep yourself out of the kitchen, consider this trick: stuff a backpack with rocks and wear it. It will literally weigh you down, helping you to consider the consequences of your actions. In one study, students who wore 15 pound backpacks were more likely to choose healthy snacks than were students who wore much lighter backpacks.

See Your Future Abs. Create a vision board. On it, list the reasons you are running for abs, especially reasons that go *beyond* pure vanity. For example, a slimmer body is easier to propel through space, making running feel even more blissful. Depending on your current waist circumference, ditching belly fat may also halve your risk of heart disease as well as slash your risk of dementia, breast cancer, and colon cancer.

Listen to Music. The faster the beat, the faster you'll run. Music will also help you to hang on for the whole workout rather than slicing a repeat off the end.

AB-VICE

As you add more speed and hill repeats, it's easy to psyche yourself out. So split your workout into mental chunks. "Just need to do 2. Just need to do 2 more. Just need to do 1 more." It will help you to get through the workout.

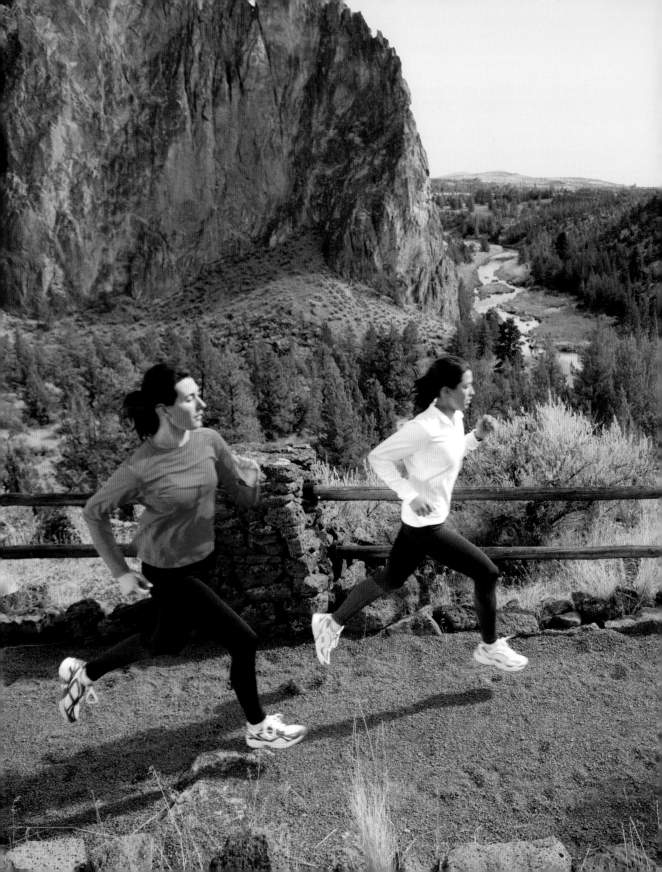

CHAPTER 6

THE RUN FOR ABS PLAN

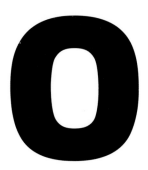**On pages** 36 to 59, you'll find a 6 week plan that will take you from ab flab to ab fab. Each day, you'll find your workout along with logs to record how you performed along with what you ate. Each week, choose your meals from the mix and match menus in chapter 7. Write down what you ate in your food journal, using the space provided.

WHAT YOU'LL NEED

This plan was made for minimalists. All you need are your running shoes, a set of dumbbells, and a heart rate monitor (optional). Try not to make the mistake of using dumbbells that a toddler could hoist. As we said earlier, going too light just doesn't challenge your muscles enough, robbing you of the afterburn that will help you to get rid of the ab flab. Choose weights that are heavy enough that you struggle to squeeze out your last rep. Then, try to increase the weight you lift every two to three weeks.

THE WORKOUTS

You'll do four workouts each week: One interval training run, one hill session, and two strength training sessions.

INTERVAL TRAINING RUN

1 X A WEEK

Intervals are short, intense efforts followed by recovery. You'll warm up by walking or jogging for 5 minutes. Then, you'll start your intervals.

During the intense part, you're pushing it, trying to get your heart rate to 85 percent of your max. Use shorter, quicker steps rather than longer steps. This will help to reduce shin splints and other aches and pains that can be triggered by faster running. Keep your feet under you and not out in front of you.

If you are brand new to running, the intense part might be a fast walk or a slow run. If you've been running for a while, it might be a sprint. What matters is your heart rate. You know you are in the intensity zone if you can only grunt and not talk. Or, put another way, you should be begging for the timer to go off, counting the seconds until you can stop.

During your recovery, run, jog or walk and catch your breath. Then do it all over again. You'll finish by cooling down by walking or jogging for 5 minutes and thanking the God of your religion that the workout is over.

As the plan progresses, you'll add more repeats and rounds as well as shorten your recovery between repeats.

During weeks 1 to 3, you'll run hard for 30 seconds followed by a 90 second recovery, for a total of 2 minutes of running. That's one round, and you'll do 5 to 8 rounds, depending on the week.

During weeks 4 to 6, you'll do a double tap progression. You'll run hard for 30 seconds and recover for 30 seconds three times, for a total of three minutes of running. That's one round. Then you'll rest for 90 seconds. Then you'll repeat the whole sequence up to 6 times, depending on the week.

	INTENSE RUNNING TIME @ 85 PERCENT HR	RECOVERY TIME @ 70 PERCENT HR	# of REPEATS	# of ROUNDS	TOTAL RUNNING TIME (not including warmup/cool down)
WEEK 1	30 seconds	90 seconds	0	5-6	10-12 min
WEEK 2	30 seconds	90 seconds	0	6-7	12-14 min
WEEK 3	30 seconds	90 seconds	0	7-8	14-16 min
WEEK 4	30 seconds	30 seconds	3 x	4-5	18-22 min
WEEK 5	30 seconds	30 seconds	3 x	5-6	22-27 min
WEEK 6	30 seconds	30 seconds	3 x	6-7	27-31 min

HILLS

1 X A WEEK

Hills enhance running form by increasing knee lift, improve joint mobility, strengthen your legs and torch calories.

Look for a hill that's a 5 to 8 percent grade. If you live in a flat area, look for bridges, parking garages, or just use a treadmill set to a 5 to 8 percent grade.

Start with a 5-minute walk or jog to warm up.

Then depending on your level of fitness, walk, jog or run up the hill for 30 seconds. How fast you run depends on how fast you can run. Again, as with the intervals, let your heart rate be your guide. Whether you are walking, jogging or sprinting uphill, you want to hit 85% of your max heart rate. Then walk down the hill and rest for 90 seconds, until your heart rate returns to 70% of your max. Then tackle the hill again... and again....and again, for the specified number of rounds.

Once you've completed your rounds, cool down by walking or running slowly for 5 minutes. Increase the number of hills each week.

Week 1 = 4-5 rounds
Week 2 = 6-7 rounds
Week 3 = 7-8 rounds
Week 4 = 8-9 rounds
Week 5 = 9-10 rounds
Week 6 = 10 rounds

STRENGTH TRAINING

2 X A WEEK

Your Abs Circuit includes the six exercises on pages 28 to 33. All six moves count as one circuit. Do all six moves one after the other, resting for 30 to 45 seconds between exercises. After completing the last movement, rest for 2 to 3 minutes. Every two to three weeks, make at least 2 to 3 exercises harder than the week before by lifting a heavier weight or using an advanced option.

During weeks 1 to 3, do two circuits. Do three circuits for weeks 4 to 6.

As the exercises get easier follow the progressions listed for each exercise. Go into each workout with fresh legs. Don't run first. If you crave a run, treat yourself a short 1-3 mile fast run afterward (and not before).

Plank

Use this ultimate core exercises to work your abdominal muscles and stabilize your core.

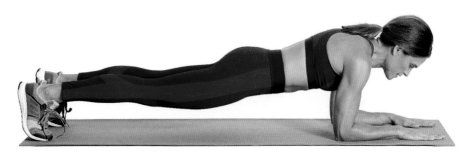

Lie face down with your elbows under your shoulders and hands face down. Grip the floor with your hands. Lift your hips, bringing your head, upper back, hips and heels into a straight line, with your core engaged.

Hold for 30 seconds.

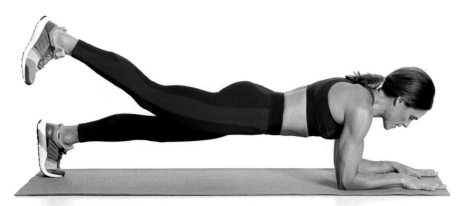

Once you can easily hold for 30 seconds, progress to lifting one leg slightly off the floor for 3 to 5 seconds. Then lift the other leg. Perform 4 to 5 lifts on each side.

Hip and Thigh Extension

This exercise will get your legs and glutes firing while also working your core.

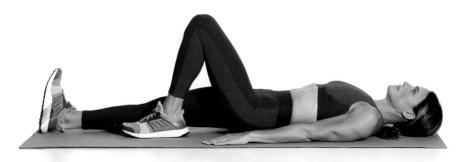

Lie on your back with your left leg bent and left foot firmly planted. Extend your right leg.

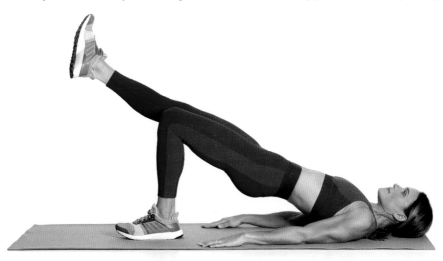

Drive through the heel of the left foot to lift your hips and right leg while maintaining core stability. Lower and repeat for a total of 8 to 10 reps. Then switch legs.

Progression: To make the move harder, hold for 3-5 seconds at the top.

Front Squat

Compound movements like a Front Squat are key to burning tons of calories and getting your metabolism up.

Stand tall with your feet shoulder-width apart. Hold a dumbbell or Kettlebell with both hands in front of your body at chest height with elbows bent in close to your body.

Squat until your thighs are at or below parallel to the floor. Return to the starting position. Keep your knees tracking over your toes and keep your heels down the entire time. Complete 8 to 10 reps.

Progression: As the exercise gets easier, switch to a heavier dumbbell.

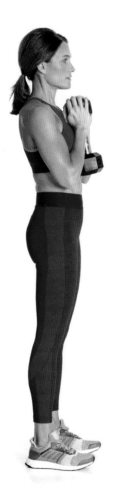
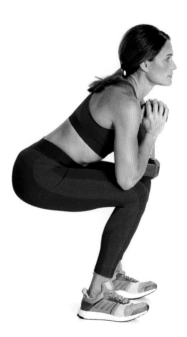

Single Arm Dumbbell Push Press

Anytime you press a weight overhead, your core will get a workout. This exercise works your upper body, lower body, and your core.

Stand tall with your feet shoulder-width apart. Hold a dumbbell in your left hand at your shoulder.

Bend your legs as if you are getting ready to jump.

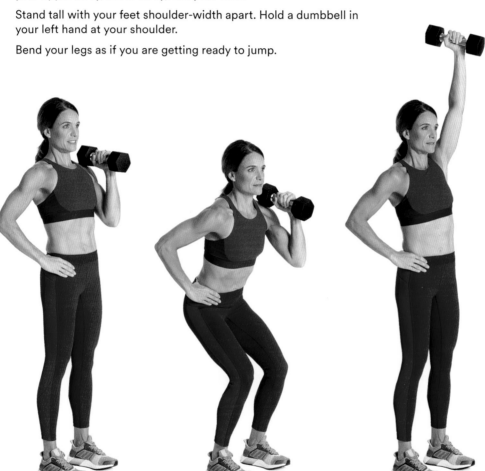

Using the power of your legs, drive the weight up overhead to land in a locked-out position with a straight arm and core engaged.

Lower the weight carefully and repeat for a total of 8 to 10 reps. Then switch sides.

Progression: As the exercise gets easier, switch to a heavier dumbbell.

Dumbbell Reverse Lunge with Offset Load

Whenever you hold a dumbbell only in one hand, your core must work harder to stabilize your body.

Stand tall with your feet hip-width apart. Hold a dumbbell in your right hand at your side.

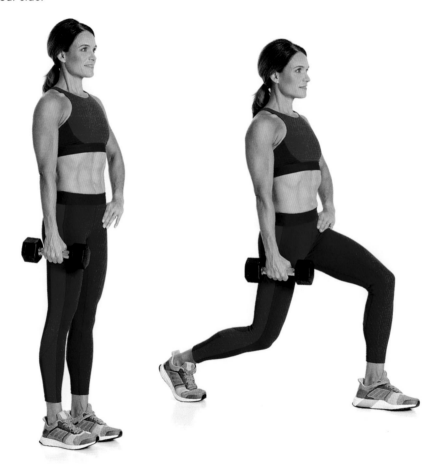

Keeping your upper body upright and core tight, shift your weight to your left foot and step backward with the right foot. Drop your hips and the back knee into a lunge. Then drive back up through the left heel and return to the starting position. Do 8 to 10 reps. Then switch sides.

Progression: Switch to a heavier dumbbell as the exercise gets easy.

Dumbbell Bent Over Row

You can't have abs without great posture, and this exercise will help you with just that.

Grab two dumbbells. As if you were completing a deadlift, bend forward until your torso is parallel to the floor, with your back straight and arms hanging down.

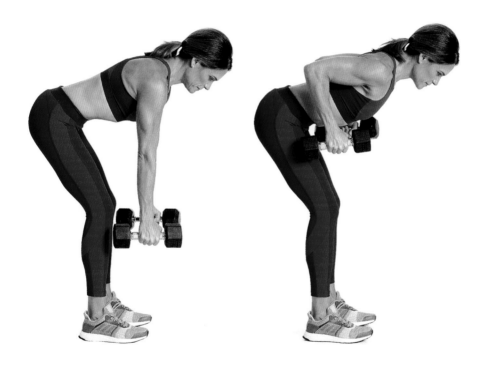

Using your upper back, pull your shoulder blades back and toward each other. Bend your elbows to row the dumbbells up to your sides. Pause, then return to the starting position. Do 8 to 10 reps.

Progression: Use a heavier dumbbell as the exercise gets easy.

THE POST CIRCUIT RUN

After making your strength training the priority you have the option to head out on a short, fast run. Find a flat loop or out and back that you can repeat each week. Time yourself to improve your speed week after week.

A Few Final Pointers

For best results, use this advice.

Go at *your* pace. If you are a beginner, do a combination of walking and slow running for your intervals and hills. As your fitness improves, do less walking and more running. Let your heart rate guide you. Aim to get it to 85 percent of your max heart rate on the hills and fast intervals and then recover at 70 percent. Not sure how to calculate your max heart rate? See the next tip.

Consider investing in a heart rate monitor. These handy devices can help ensure your intensity reaches 85% of your max heart rate for the work periods. They'll also help to ensure you are fully recovered to 70% of your max heart rate before you tackle your next repeat.

To figure out your target heart rate, use these simple equations:
- 220 – Your Age = Max Heart Rate
- Max Heart Rate x 0.85 = 85% of Max Heart Rate (work interval)
- Max Heart Rate x 0.70 = 70% of Max Heart Rate (recovery target)

These are estimates, and you may need to adjust them as you go. To determine the accuracy of the equations, check how you feel.
- Below 70% = Can sing a song
- 70–85% = Can talk, but only in 2 or 3 word sentences
- 85% or higher = Can't talk. Only grunt.

AB-VICE

Do speed work on a soft surface such as dirt, grass, or a spongy track to reduce the impact of a hard session. You'll be able to train harder and recover faster.

Don't run before strength training.
You want fresh arms and legs so you can really push yourself. If you crave more miles, though, you can run 1 to 3 miles afterward.

Don't run extra. If you're used to doing a lot of distance, it might feel unnatural to run only a few miles at a time, but lower mileage is so important to your recovery and your overall success. Give it 6 weeks. If the results don't make you a believer by then, but all means, extend your runs. Until then, pour all of your stress into your intensity. Rather than run farther, run faster.

Weigh yourself once a week.
Weight can fluctuate wildly from day to day. Once a week weigh ins will give you a better gauge on your progress than daily ones. Even better than tracking your weight, consider taking your measurements. You may find that your waist circumference shrinks, even as your weight stays the same. This is a sign that you are replacing fat with muscle, which is heavier than fat.

Get creative with your record keeping. In the plan, you'll find space to record your reps, sets, meals and other details, but feel absolutely welcome to add your own personal flair to your record keeping. For example, Olympic medalist Deena Kastor records the basic details of her workouts, "But when I've run really well or felt great, I shade those boxes on the calendar with a pink high-lighter and add more details," she says. "I write down something that will bring back the emotions – how I drove my knees up a long hill, or felt I could have run with the best in the world that day. Then just before I go out to do the same workout the next time, I read what's in the pink box. It builds my confidence and helps me visualize how to do it again." Consider doing the same with your log.

 COMMIT TO ABS

At this point, one of three things is true for you.

1. You were ready to Run for Abs when you bought this guide and you just want to get started on the program already.

2. You weren't quite sold when you bought this guide, but you are now.

3. You're not yet on board, and nothing we tell you is going to get you there.

If #3 is true for you, we've like to ask you something. Has your current running strategy been working for you? Assuming we're right and the answer to that question is no, then we'd like you to consider the advice of Rachel Cosgrove, CSCS, the coach who designed the Run for Abs workouts. Just give it a try. Commit to Run for Abs for six weeks. See what happens. What do you have to lose other than your stubborn belly fat?

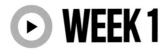

WEEK 1

Set yourself up for success. Take a look at your calendar and schedule in these workouts. Turn to chapter 7 and pick the meals you will eat for the week. Pencil them into the "Eat for Abs" chart, in the space provided. Based on those meals, hit the grocery store and stock up on what you need.

RUN FOR ABS

Day 1	Day 2	Day 3	Day 4	Day 5	Day 6	Day 7
Strength 2 Circuits Fast Run 1-3 miles	Off	Intervals 30s Hard 90s Recovery 5-6 Rounds	Strength 2 Circuits Fast Run 1-3 miles	Off	Hills 30s Uphill 90s Recovery 4-5 Rounds	Off

EAT FOR ABS

	Day 1	Day 2	Day 3	Day 4	Day 5	Day 6	Day 7
Breakfast							
Lunch							
Dinner							
Snacks							

Day 1

DATE:_____   ▶ MY WEIGHT:_____

STRENGTH TRAINING + OPTIONAL SHORT, FAST RUN

☐ **Plank** _____ seconds
(Goal = at least 30)

☐ **Hip/Thigh Extension**
_____ Reps
(Goal = 8-10 on each side)

☐ **Front Squat**
_____ Reps *(Goal = 8-10)*

☐ **Single Arm Dumbbell Push Press**
_____ Reps *(Goal = 8-10)* _____ Weight

☐ **Dumbbell Reverse Lunge with offset load**
_____ Reps *(Goal = 8-10)* _____ Weight

☐ **Dumbbell Bent Over Row** _____
Reps *(Goal = 8-10)* _____ Weight

Sets: _____ *(Goal = 2)*
Optional short, fast run: _____ Miles *(Goal = 1-3)* _____ Time

Breakfast

Lunch

Dinner

Notes:

Day 2

DATE:_____

☐ RECOVER, RELAX, RESTORE

Breakfast

Lunch

Dinner

Notes:

Day 3   DATE:_____

☐ INTERVAL TRAINING RUN

1. Warm up by walking or running slowly for 5 minutes.

2. Sprint, run, or walk as hard as you can for 30 seconds, aiming to get your heart rate up to 85 percent of your max.

3. Recover (walk/jog) for 90 seconds, allowing your heart rate to drop down to 70 percent of your max.

4. Repeat steps 2 & 3 for a total of 5 to 6 rounds.

5. Cool down by walking or running slowly for 5 minutes.

Rounds completed: _____ *(Goal = 5-6)*

WHAT I ATE

Breakfast

Lunch

Dinner

Notes:

Day 4   DATE:_____

THE WORKOUT

STRENGTH TRAINING + OPTIONAL SHORT, FAST RUN

☐ **Plank** _____ seconds
(Goal = at least 30)

☐ **Hip/Thigh Extension**
_____ Reps
(Goal = 8-10 on each side)

☐ **Front Squat**
_____ Reps *(Goal = 8-10)*

☐ **Single Arm Dumbbell Push Press**
_____ Reps *(Goal = 8-10)* _____ Weight

☐ **Dumbbell Reverse Lunge with offset load**
_____ Reps *(Goal = 8-10)* _____ Weight

☐ **Dumbbell Bent Over Row**
_____ Reps *(Goal = 8-10)* _____ Weight

Sets:_____ *(Goal = 2)*
Optional short, fast run: _____ Miles *(Goal = 1-3)* _____ Time

WHAT I ATE

Breakfast

Lunch

Dinner

Notes:

Day 5   DATE:_____

☐ **RECOVER, RELAX, RESTORE**

WHAT I ATE

Breakfast

Lunch

Dinner

Notes:

Day 6   DATE:_____

THE WORKOUT

☐ **HILL REPEAT RUN**

1. Walk or run slowly for 5 minutes to warm up.

2. Walk or run up a steep hill for 30 seconds, getting your heart rate to 85 percent of your max.

3. Walk down the hill.

4. Recover for 90 seconds, until your heart rate returns to 70 percent of your max.

5. Repeat steps 2-4 for a total of 4 to 5 rounds.

6. Cool down by walking or running slowly for five minutes.

Rounds completed: _____ *(Goal = 4-5)*

WHAT I ATE

Breakfast

Lunch

Dinner

Notes:

Day 7   DATE:_____

THE WORKOUT

☐ **RECOVER, RELAX, RESTORE**

WHAT I ATE

Breakfast

Lunch

Dinner

Notes:

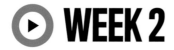

WEEK 2

Don't forget to plan ahead. Take a look at your calendar and schedule in these workouts. Turn to chapter 7 and pick the meals you will eat for the week. Pencil them into the "Eat for Abs" chart. Make a list and head to the grocery store to ensure you have everything you need.

RUN FOR ABS

Day 8	Day 9	Day 10	Day 11	Day 12	Day 13	Day 14
Strength 2 Circuits Fast Run 1-3 miles	Off	Intervals 30s Hard 90s Recovery 6-7 Rounds	Strength 2 Circuits Fast Run 1-3 miles	Off	Hills 30s Uphill 90s Recovery 6-7 Rounds	Off

EAT FOR ABS

	Day 8	Day 9	Day 10	Day 11	Day 12	Day 13	Day 14
Breakfast							
Lunch							
Dinner							
Snacks							

Day 8 DATE:_____

▶ MY WEIGHT:_____

STRENGTH TRAINING + OPTIONAL SHORT, FAST RUN

☐ **Plank** _____ seconds
(Goal = at least 30)

☐ **Hip/Thigh Extension**
_____ Reps
(Goal = 8-10 on each side)

☐ **Front Squat**
_____ Reps *(Goal = 8-10)*

☐ **Single Arm Dumbbell Push Press**
_____ Reps *(Goal = 8-10)* _____ Weight

☐ **Dumbbell Reverse Lunge with offset load**
_____ Reps *(Goal = 8-10)* _____ Weight

☐ **Dumbbell Bent Over Row**
_____ Reps *(Goal = 8-10)* _____ Weight

Sets: _____ *(Goal = 2)*
Optional short, fast run: _____ Miles *(Goal = 1-3)* _____ Time

WHAT I ATE

Breakfast

Lunch

Dinner

Notes:

Day 9 DATE:_____

THE WORKOUT

☐ RECOVER, RELAX, RESTORE

WHAT I ATE

Breakfast

Lunch

Dinner

Notes:

Day 10   DATE:_____

THE WORKOUT

☐ **INTERVAL TRAINING RUN**

1. Warm up by walking or running slowly for 5 minutes.

2. Sprint, run, or walk as hard as you can for 30 seconds, aiming to get your heart rate up to 85 percent of your max.

3. Recover (walk/jog) for 90 seconds, allowing your heart rate to drop down to 70 percent of your max.

4. Repeat steps 2 & 3 for a total of 6 to 7 rounds.

5. Cool down by walking or running slowly for 5 minutes.

Rounds completed: _____ (Goal = 6-7)

WHAT I ATE

Breakfast

Lunch

Dinner

Notes:

Day 11   DATE:_____

THE WORKOUT

STRENGTH TRAINING + OPTIONAL SHORT, FAST RUN

☐ **Plank** _____ seconds
(Goal = at least 30)

☐ **Hip/Thigh Extension**
_____ Reps
(Goal = 8-10 on each side)

☐ **Front Squat**
_____ Reps (Goal = 8-10)

☐ **Single Arm Dumbbell Push Press**
_____ Reps (Goal = 8-10) _____ Weight

☐ **Dumbbell Reverse Lunge with offset load**
_____ Reps (Goal = 8-10) _____ Weight

☐ **Dumbbell Bent Over Row**
_____ Reps (Goal = 8-10) _____ Weight

Sets:_____ (Goal = 2)
Optional short, fast run: _____ Miles (Goal = 1-3) _____ Time

WHAT I ATE

Breakfast

Lunch

Dinner

Notes:

Day 12   DATE:_____

☐ **RECOVER, RELAX, RESTORE**

WHAT I ATE

Breakfast

Lunch

Dinner

Notes:

Day 13   DATE:_____

THE WORKOUT

☐ **HILL REPEAT RUN**

1. Walk or run slowly for 5 minutes to warm up.

2. Walk or run up a steep hill for 30 seconds, getting your heart rate to 85 percent of your max.

3. Walk down the hill.

4. Recover for 90 seconds, until your heart rate returns to 70 percent of your max.

5. Repeat steps 2-4 for a total of 6 to 7 rounds.

6. Cool down by walking or running slowly for five minutes.

Rounds completed: _____ *(Goal = 6-7)*

WHAT I ATE

Breakfast

Lunch

Dinner

Notes:

Day 14   DATE:_____

THE WORKOUT

☐ **RECOVER, RELAX, RESTORE**

WHAT I ATE

Breakfast

Lunch

Dinner

Notes:

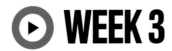 # WEEK 3

Schedule these workouts into your calendar and pick your week's meals from chapter 7. Write them in the space provided in the "Eat for Abs" chart.

RUN FOR ABS

Day 15	Day 16	Day 17	Day 18	Day 19	Day 20	Day 21
Strength 2 Circuits Fast Run 1-3 miles	Off	Intervals 30s Hard 90s Recovery 7-8 Rounds	Strength 2 Circuits Fast Run 1-3 miles	Off	Hills 30s Uphill 90s Recovery 7-8 Rounds	Off

EAT FOR ABS

	Day 15	Day 16	Day 17	Day 18	Day 19	Day 20	Day 21
Breakfast							
Lunch							
Dinner							
Snacks							

Day 15   DATE:_____   ▶ MY WEIGHT:_____

STRENGTH TRAINING + OPTIONAL SHORT, FAST RUN

☐ **Plank** _____ seconds
(Goal = at least 30)

☐ **Hip/Thigh Extension**
_____ Reps
(Goal = 8-10 on each side)

☐ **Front Squat**
_____ Reps *(Goal = 8-10)*

☐ **Single Arm Dumbbell Push Press**
_____ Reps *(Goal = 8-10)* _____ Weight

☐ **Dumbbell Reverse Lunge with offset load**
_____ Reps *(Goal = 8-10)* _____ Weight

☐ **Dumbbell Bent Over Row**
_____ Reps *(Goal = 8-10)* _____ Weight

Sets:_____ *(Goal = 2)*
Optional short, fast run: _____ Miles *(Goal = 1-3)* _____ Time

WHAT I ATE

Breakfast

Lunch

Dinner

Notes:

Day 16   DATE:_____

THE WORKOUT

☐ **RECOVER, RELAX, RESTORE**

WHAT I ATE

Breakfast

Lunch

Dinner

Notes:

Day 17   DATE:_____

☐ INTERVAL TRAINING RUN

1. Warm up by walking or running slowly for 5 minutes.

2. Sprint, run, or walk as hard as you can for 30 seconds, aiming to get your heart rate up to 85 percent of your max.

3. Recover (walk/jog) for 90 seconds, allowing your heart rate to drop down to 70 percent of your max.

4. Repeat steps 2 & 3 for a total of 7 to 8 rounds.

5. Cool down by walking or running slowly for 5 minutes.

Rounds completed: _____ *(Goal = 7-8)*

WHAT I ATE

Breakfast

Lunch

Dinner

Notes:

Day 18   DATE:_____

THE WORKOUT

STRENGTH TRAINING + OPTIONAL SHORT, FAST RUN

☐ **Plank** _____ seconds
(Goal = at least 30)

☐ **Hip/Thigh Extension**
_____ Reps
(Goal = 8-10 on each side)

☐ **Front Squat**
_____ Reps *(Goal = 8-10)*

☐ **Single Arm Dumbbell Push Press**
_____ Reps *(Goal = 8-10)* _____ Weight

☐ **Dumbbell Reverse Lunge with offset load**
_____ Reps *(Goal = 8-10)* _____ Weight

☐ **Dumbbell Bent Over Row**
_____ Reps *(Goal = 8-10)* _____ Weight

Sets: _____ *(Goal = 2)*
Optional short, fast run: _____ Miles *(Goal = 1-3)* _____ Time

WHAT I ATE

Breakfast

Lunch

Dinner

Notes:

Day 19   DATE:_____

☐ **RECOVER, RELAX, RESTORE**

WHAT I ATE

Breakfast

Lunch

Dinner

Notes:

Day 20   DATE:_____

THE WORKOUT

☐ **HILL REPEAT RUN**

1. Walk or run slowly for 5 minutes to warm up.

2. Walk or run up a steep hill for 30 seconds, getting your heart rate to 85 percent of your max.

3. Walk down the hill.

4. Recover for 90 seconds, until your heart rate returns to 70 percent of your max.

5. Repeat steps 2-4 for a total of 7 to 8 rounds.

6. Cool down by walking or running slowly for five minutes.

Rounds completed: _____ *(Goal = 7-8)*

WHAT I ATE

Breakfast

Lunch

Dinner

Notes:

Day 21   DATE:_____

THE WORKOUT

☐ **RECOVER, RELAX, RESTORE**

WHAT I ATE

Breakfast

Lunch

Dinner

Notes:

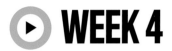

WEEK 4

Your workouts get a little longer this week. Make sure to plan for that. Also, don't forget to plan and prep your meals, writing them in the space provided.

RUN FOR ABS

Day 22	Day 23	Day 24	Day 25	Day 26	Day 27	Day 28
Strength 3 Circuits Fast Run 1-3 miles	Off	Intervals 30s Hard 30s Recovery 3 Repeats, followed by 90s recovery 4-5 Rounds	Strength 3 Circuits Fast Run 1-3 miles	Off	Hills 30s Uphill 90s Recovery 8-9 Rounds	Off

EAT FOR ABS

	Day 22	Day 23	Day 24	Day 25	Day 26	Day 27	Day 28
Breakfast							
Lunch							
Dinner							
Snacks							

Day 22 DATE:_____ ▶ MY WEIGHT:_____

STRENGTH TRAINING + OPTIONAL SHORT, FAST RUN

☐ **Plank** _____ seconds
  (Goal = at least 30)

☐ **Hip/Thigh Extension**
  _____ Reps
  (Goal = 8-10 on each side)

☐ **Front Squat**
  _____ Reps *(Goal = 8-10)*

☐ **Single Arm Dumbbell Push Press**
  _____ Reps *(Goal = 8-10)* _____ Weight

☐ **Dumbbell Reverse Lunge with offset load**
  _____ Reps *(Goal = 8-10)* _____ Weight

☐ **Dumbbell Bent Over Row** _____
  Reps *(Goal = 8-10)* _____ Weight

Sets: _____ *(Goal = 3)*
Optional short, fast run: _____ Miles *(Goal = 1-3)* _____ Time

WHAT I ATE

Breakfast

Lunch

Dinner

Notes:

Day 23 DATE:_____

THE WORKOUT

☐ RECOVER, RELAX, RESTORE

WHAT I ATE

Breakfast

Lunch

Dinner

Notes:

Day 24 DATE:_____

☐ INTERVAL TRAINING RUN

NOTE: This week, shorten your recovery to just 30 seconds between fast bouts.

1. Warm up by walking or running slowly for 5 minutes.

2. Sprint, run, or walk as hard as you can for 30 seconds, aiming to get your heart rate up to 85 percent of your max.

3. Recover (walk/jog) for 30 seconds, allowing your heart rate to drop down to 70 percent of your max.

4. Repeat steps 2 & 3 three times.

5. Recover 90 seconds.

6. Repeat steps 2-5 for a total of four to five rounds.

7. Cool down by walking or running slowly for 5 minutes.

Rounds completed: _____ *(Goal = 4-5)*

WHAT I ATE

Breakfast

Lunch

Dinner

Notes:

Day 25 DATE:_____

THE WORKOUT

STRENGTH TRAINING + OPTIONAL SHORT, FAST RUN

☐ **Plank** _____ seconds
(Goal = at least 30)

☐ **Hip/Thigh Extension**
_____ Reps
(Goal = 8-10 on each side)

☐ **Front Squat**
_____ Reps *(Goal = 8-10)*

☐ **Single Arm Dumbbell Push Press**
_____ Reps *(Goal = 8-10)* _____ Weight

☐ **Dumbbell Reverse Lunge with offset load**
_____ Reps *(Goal = 8-10)* _____ Weight

☐ **Dumbbell Bent Over Row**
_____ Reps *(Goal = 8-10)* _____ Weight

Sets:_____ *(Goal = 3)*
Optional short, fast run: _____ Miles *(Goal = 1-3)* _____ Time

WHAT I ATE

Breakfast

Lunch

Dinner

Notes:

Day 26   DATE:_____

THE WORKOUT

☐ **RECOVER, RELAX, RESTORE**

WHAT I ATE

Breakfast

Lunch

Dinner

Notes:

Day 27   DATE:_____

THE WORKOUT

☐ **HILL REPEAT RUN**

1. Walk or run slowly for 5 minutes to warm up.

2. Walk or run up a steep hill for 30 seconds, getting your heart rate to 85 percent of your max.

3. Walk down the hill.

4. Recover for 90 seconds, until your heart rate returns to 70 percent of your max.

5. Repeat steps 2-4 for a total of 8-9 rounds.

6. Cool down by walking or running slowly for five minutes.

Rounds completed: _____ *(Goal = 8-9)*

WHAT I ATE

Breakfast

Lunch

Dinner

Notes:

Day 28   DATE:_____

THE WORKOUT

☐ **RECOVER, RELAX, RESTORE**

WHAT I ATE

Breakfast

Lunch

Dinner

Notes:

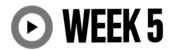 # WEEK 5

Use these charts to plan your week. Don't forget to plan your meals, jotting them down in the space provided.

RUN FOR ABS

Day 29	Day 30	Day 31	Day 32	Day 33	Day 34	Day 35
Strength 3 Circuits Fast Run 1-3 miles	Off	Intervals 30s Hard 30s Recovery 3 Repeats, followed by 90s recovery 5-6 Rounds	Strength 3 Circuits Fast Run 1-3 miles	Off	Hills 30s Uphill 90s Recovery 9-10 Rounds	Off

EAT FOR ABS

	Day 29	Day 30	Day 31	Day 32	Day 33	Day 34	Day 35
Breakfast							
Lunch							
Dinner							
Snacks							

Day 29 DATE:_____ ▶ MY WEIGHT:_____

STRENGTH TRAINING + OPTIONAL SHORT, FAST RUN

☐ **Plank** _____ seconds
(Goal = at least 30)

☐ **Hip/Thigh Extension**
_____ Reps
(Goal = 8-10 on each side)

☐ **Front Squat**
_____ Reps *(Goal = 8-10)*

☐ **Single Arm Dumbbell Push Press**
_____ Reps *(Goal = 8-10)* _____ Weight

☐ **Dumbbell Reverse Lunge with offset load**
_____ Reps *(Goal = 8-10)* _____ Weight

☐ **Dumbbell Bent Over Row**
_____ Reps *(Goal = 8-10)* _____ Weight

Sets: _____ *(Goal = 3)*
Optional short, fast run: _____ Miles *(Goal = 1-3)* _____ Time

Breakfast

Lunch

Dinner

Notes:

Day 30 DATE:_____

☐ RECOVER, RELAX, RESTORE

Breakfast

Lunch

Dinner

Notes:

Day 31   DATE:_____

☐ INTERVAL TRAINING RUN

1. Warm up by walking or running slowly for 5 minutes.

2. Sprint, run, or walk as hard as you can for 30 seconds, aiming to get your heart rate up to 85 percent of your max.

3. Recover (walk/jog) for 30 seconds, allowing your heart rate to drop down to 70 percent of your max.

4. Repeat steps 2 & 3 three times.

5. Recover 90 seconds.

6. Repeat steps 2-5 for a total of five to six rounds.

7. Cool down by walking or running slowly for 5 minutes.

Rounds completed:_____ *(Goal = 5-6)*

WHAT I ATE

Breakfast

Lunch

Dinner

Notes:

Day 32   DATE:_____

THE WORKOUT

STRENGTH TRAINING + OPTIONAL SHORT, FAST RUN

☐ **Plank** _____ seconds
(Goal = at least 30)

☐ **Hip/Thigh Extension**
_____ Reps
(Goal = 8-10 on each side)

☐ **Front Squat**
_____ Reps *(Goal = 8-10)*

☐ **Single Arm Dumbbell Push Press**
_____ Reps *(Goal = 8-10)* _____ Weight

☐ **Dumbbell Reverse Lunge with offset load**
_____ Reps *(Goal = 8-10)* _____ Weight

☐ **Dumbbell Bent Over Row**
_____ Reps *(Goal = 8-10)* _____ Weight

Sets:_____ *(Goal = 3)*
Optional short, fast run: _____ Miles *(Goal = 1-3)* _____ Time

WHAT I ATE

Breakfast

Lunch

Dinner

Notes:

Day 33   DATE:_____

☐ **RECOVER, RELAX, RESTORE**

WHAT I ATE

Breakfast

Lunch

Dinner

Notes:

Day 34   DATE:_____

THE WORKOUT

☐ **HILL REPEAT RUN**

1. Walk or run slowly for 5 minutes to warm up.

2. Walk or run up a steep hill for 30 seconds, getting your heart rate to 85 percent of your max.

3. Walk down the hill.

4. Recover for 90 seconds, until your heart rate returns to 70 percent of your max.

5. Repeat steps 2-4 for a total of 9-10 rounds.

6. Cool down by walking or running slowly for five minutes.

Rounds completed: _____ *(Goal = 9-10)*

WHAT I ATE

Breakfast

Lunch

Dinner

Notes:

Day 35   DATE:_____

THE WORKOUT

☐ **RECOVER, RELAX, RESTORE**

WHAT I ATE

Breakfast

Lunch

Dinner

Notes:

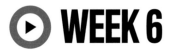 # WEEK 6

You're almost done. We hope your abs are starting to show! Remember to plan ahead. Choose your meals from chapter 7, and write them down in the space provided.

RUN FOR ABS

Day 36	Day 37	Day 38	Day 39	Day 40	Day 41	Day 42
Strength 3 Circuits Fast Run 1-3 miles	Off	Intervals 30s Hard 30s Recovery 3 Repeats, followed by 90s recovery 6-7 Rounds	Strength 3 Circuits Fast Run 1-3 miles	Off	Hills 30s Uphill 90s Recovery 10 Rounds	Off

EAT FOR ABS

	Day 36	Day 37	Day 38	Day 39	Day 40	Day 41	Day 42
Breakfast							
Lunch							
Dinner							
Snacks							

Day 36   DATE:_____   ▶ MY WEIGHT:_____

STRENGTH TRAINING + OPTIONAL SHORT, FAST RUN

☐ **Plank** _____ seconds
(Goal = at least 30)

☐ **Hip/Thigh Extension**
_____ Reps
(Goal = 8-10 on each side)

☐ **Front Squat**
_____ Reps *(Goal = 8-10)*

☐ **Single Arm Dumbbell Push Press**
_____ Reps *(Goal = 8-10)* _____ Weight

☐ **Dumbbell Reverse Lunge with offset load**
_____ Reps *(Goal = 8-10)* _____ Weight

☐ **Dumbbell Bent Over Row**
_____ Reps *(Goal = 8-10)* _____ Weight

Sets: _____ *(Goal = 3)*
Optional short, fast run: _____ Miles *(Goal = 1-3)* _____ Time

WHAT I ATE

Breakfast

Lunch

Dinner

Notes:

Day 37   DATE:_____

THE WORKOUT

☐ **RECOVER, RELAX, RESTORE**

WHAT I ATE

Breakfast

Lunch

Dinner

Notes:

Day 38   DATE:_____

☐ INTERVAL TRAINING RUN

1. Warm up by walking or running slowly for 5 minutes.

2. Sprint, run, or walk as hard as you can for 30 seconds, aiming to get your heart rate up to 85 percent of your max.

3. Recover (walk/jog) for 30 seconds, allowing your heart rate to drop down to 70 percent of your max.

4. Repeat steps 2 & 3 three times

5. Recover 90 seconds.

6. Repeat steps 2-5 for a total of six to seven rounds.

7. Cool down by walking or running slowly for 5 minutes.

Intervals: _____ *(Goal = 6-7)*

WHAT I ATE

Breakfast

Lunch

Dinner

Notes:

Day 39   DATE:_____

THE WORKOUT

STRENGTH TRAINING + OPTIONAL SHORT, FAST RUN

☐ **Plank** _____ seconds
(Goal = at least 30)

☐ **Hip/Thigh Extension**
_____ Reps
(Goal = 8-10 on each side)

☐ **Front Squat**
_____ Reps *(Goal = 8-10)*

☐ **Single Arm Dumbbell Push Press**
_____ Reps *(Goal = 8-10)* _____ Weight

☐ **Dumbbell Reverse Lunge with offset load**
_____ Reps *(Goal = 8-10)* _____ Weight

☐ **Dumbbell Bent Over Row**
_____ Reps *(Goal = 8-10)* _____ Weight

Sets: _____ *(Goal = 3)*
Optional short, fast run: _____ Miles *(Goal = 1-3)* _____ Time

WHAT I ATE

Breakfast

Lunch

Dinner

Notes:

Day 40   DATE:_____

☐ **RECOVER, RELAX, RESTORE**

WHAT I ATE

Breakfast

Lunch

Dinner

Notes:

Day 41   DATE:_____

THE WORKOUT

☐ **HILL REPEAT RUN**

1. Warm up by walking or running slowly for 5 minutes.

2. Walk or run up a steep hill for 30 seconds, getting your heart rate to 85 percent of your max.

3. Walk back down.

4. Recover for 90 seconds, until your heart rate returns to 70 percent of your max.

5. Repeat steps 2-4 for a total of 10 rounds.

6. Walk or run slowly for 5 minutes to cool down.

Rounds completed: _____ *(Goal = 10)*

WHAT I ATE

Breakfast

Lunch

Dinner

Notes:

Day 42   DATE:_____

THE WORKOUT

☐ **RECOVER, RELAX, RESTORE**

WHAT I ATE

Breakfast

Lunch

Dinner

Notes:

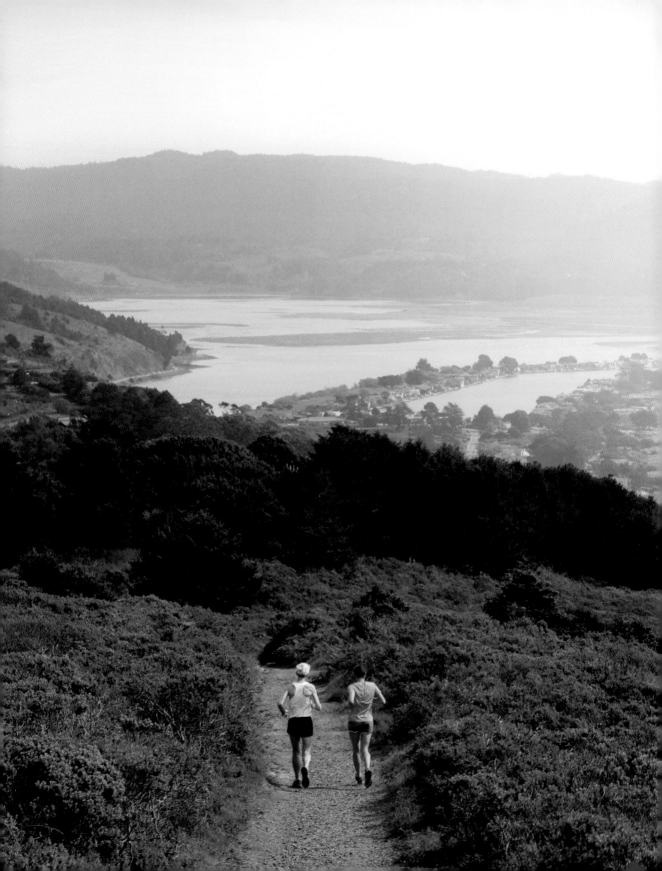

CHAPTER 7

THE RUN FOR ABS MENUS

Nutrition expert Erin Palinski-Wade, RDN, worked with our test kitchen to create dozens of delicious meals that showcase the 6 Belly Fat Fighters. Each meal is already perfectly portioned for weight loss and contains the right balance of carbs, protein and fats to help you slim down without hunger. We've organized these options into breakfast, lunch, dinner and snack categories. Dig in and enjoy!

About the Menu Options

THE BELLY FAT FIGHTERS	THE MACROS	THE CALORIES
ALL MEALS AND SNACKS INCLUDE AT LEAST ONE: Lean protein Resistant starch Soluble fiber Slimming fats Fermented ingredients Anti-inflammatory spices (cayenne, turmeric, cinnamon)	**ALL MEALS AND SNACKS FALL WITHIN THESE RANGES:** 30-55% carbs 20-35% protein 25-35% fat	**THE CALORIES FOR EACH MEAL AND SNACK ROUGHLY FALL WITHIN THESE RANGES:** Breakfasts: 250-400 Lunches: 400-500 Dinners: 400-600 Snacks: 150-250 Daily totals: 1200-1750

▶ BREAKFASTS

62 Avocado Egg Breakfast Sandwich

62 Greek Yogurt Parfait

63 Power Up Pancakes with Yogurt and Berries

63 Avocado Toast

63 Berry Cinnamon Overnight Oatmeal

64 Green Lentil Smoothie

64 Spicy Spinach Frittata Muffins

AVOCADO EGG BREAKFAST SANDWICH

PREP TIME: 3 minutes
TOTAL TIME: 5 minutes
Makes 1 serving

Top a slice of multigrain toast with ¼ sliced avocado, 2 scrambled eggs, and a pinch of salt and cayenne pepper. Top with another slice of toast and cut in half.

NUTRITION (*per serving*): 381 calories, 21 g protein, 34 g carbohydrates, 8 g fiber, 5 g sugar, 19 g fat, 4 g saturated fat, 543 mg sodium

GREEK YOGURT PARFAIT

PREP TIME: 2 minutes
TOTAL TIME: 2 minutes
Makes 1 serving

In a tall glass, layer ¼ cup of walnuts, ¾ cup of blueberries, and ¾ cup of plain Greek yogurt.

NUTRITION (*per serving*): 262 calories, 21 g protein, 25 g carbohydrates, 4 g fiber, 18 g sugar, 10 g fat, 3 g saturated fat, 66 mg sodium

POWER UP PANCAKES WITH YOGURT AND BERRIES

PREP TIME: 5 minutes
TOTAL TIME: 15 minutes
Makes 2 servings

- 4 large egg whites
- 2 egg
- ¼ cup rolled oats
- ¼ cup cottage cheese
- 1 scoop vanilla protein powder
- ½ teaspoon ground cinnamon
- 2 teaspoons unsalted butter
- 1 cup fresh berries
- ¼ cup plain yogurt
- 2 teaspoons maple syrup or honey

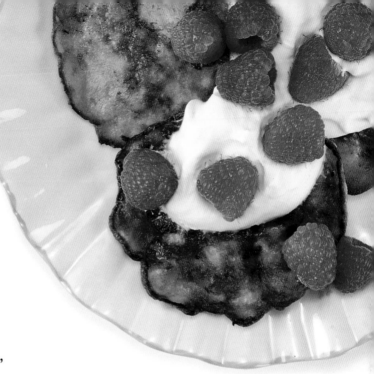

In a medium bowl whisk together the egg whites, egg, oats, cottage cheese, protein powder, and cinnamon until combined. Let sit to thicken, 5 minutes.

Heat a medium nonstick skillet over medium heat and melt the butter. Pour the batter into the skillet in 3 rounds. Cook until bubbles appear on the surface, 3 minutes. Flip and cook until golden and cooked through, 3 minutes more.

Top with berries, yogurt, and maple syrup.

NUTRITION (*per serving*): 309 calories, 32 g protein, 28 g carbohydrates, 3 g fiber, 17 g sugar, 8 g fat, 3 g saturated fat, 331 mg sodium

AVOCADO TOAST

PREP TIME: 3 minutes
TOTAL TIME: 5 minutes
Makes 1 serving

Top 1 slice of multigrain toast with ½ sliced medium avocado and ½ cup of cottage cheese.

NUTRITION (*per serving*): 287 calories, 19 g protein, 25 g carbohydrates, 5 g fiber, 5 g sugar, 15 g fat, 4 g saturated fat, 440 mg sodium

BERRY CINNAMON OVERNIGHT OATMEAL

PREP TIME: 5 minutes
TOTAL TIME: 5 minutes + overnight
Makes 2 servings

- ¾ cup rolled oats
- 1½ cup 2% milk
- ½ teaspoon ground cinnamon
  Pinch salt
- ⅔ cup fresh blueberries, raspberries, or blackberries
- 2 tablespoons toasted chopped walnuts

Divide the oatmeal, milk, cinnamon and salt among 2 pint size mason jars and stir to combine; close and refrigerate overnight.

Stir in or top with the berries and walnuts. May be eaten cold or for a warm breakfast, remove lid and microwave until warm, about 1 minute.

NUTRITION (*per serving*): 286 calories, 13 g protein, 37 g carbohydrates, 6 g fiber, 13 g sugars, 11 g fat, 3 g saturated fat, 136 mg sodium

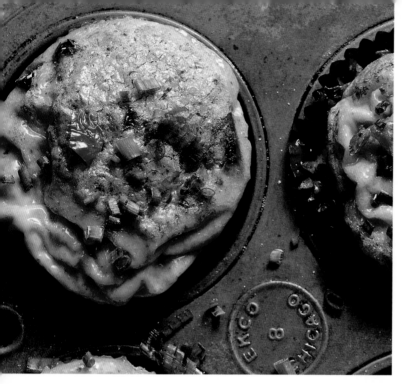

SPICY SPINACH FRITTATA MUFFINS

PREP TIME: 10 minutes
TOTAL TIME: 40 minutes
Makes 2 servings

- 2 teaspoons olive oil
- 1 small onion, finely chopped
- 2 cups baby spinach, chopped
- 1 medium tomato, chopped
- 4 eggs
- ⅓ cup shredded cheddar
- 1 tablespoon chopped fresh cilantro
- ¼ teaspoon ground cayenne
- ¼ teaspoon kosher salt

Preheat the oven to 350°F. Lightly coat an 8-cup muffin pan with cooking spray.

In a small skillet heat the oil over medium heat. Add the onion and cook, stirring until translucent, 5 minutes. Add the spinach and tomato and cook until the spinach is just wilted and the tomato juice has evaporated, 3 minutes. Remove from heat.

In a medium bowl, combine the eggs, cheese, cilantro, cayenne, and salt. Add the onion mixture and stir to combine. Divide the mixture among the muffin cups.

Bake until a wooden pick inserted in the center of one muffin comes out clean, 15 to 20 minutes. Cool the muffins on a rack for 1 minute before removing them from the pan and serving. Cool completely before storing in an airtight container in the refrigerator for up to 1 week.

NUTRITION (*per serving*): 294 calories, 18 g protein, 8 g carbohydrates, 2 g fiber, 1 g sugars, 22 g fat, 8 g saturated fat, 592 mg sodium

GREEN LENTIL SMOOTHIE

PREP TIME: 5 minutes
TOTAL TIME: 5 minutes
Makes 2 servings

- ½ medium cucumber, peeled and chopped
- 1 cup chopped kale leaves
- ½ cup cooked green lentils
- 1 frozen banana
- ½ cup cold water
- ½ cup ice
- 1 cup plain full-fat Greek yogurt
- 1 tablespoon honey
- 2 tablespoons fresh lemon juice
- 1 teaspoon flaxseed oil
- 1 teaspoon freshly grated ginger
- 1 teaspoon matcha

In a blender, combine all ingredients. Blend for 1 minute, or until smooth.

NUTRITION (*per serving*): 305 calories, 17 g protein, 43 g carbohydrates, 7 g fiber, 23 g sugar, 9 g fat, 4 g saturated fat, 57 mg sodium

▶ LUNCHES

65 Turkey Club Sandwich
65 Pepperoni Mushroom Pizza
65 Seafood Salad
66 Slow Cooker Veggie Chili
66 PB&J Parfait
67 Black Bean and Broccoli Burrito

67 Slow Cooker BBQ Pulled Chicken Salad
68 Egg Salad Wraps
68 Tuna Salad Sandwich
68 Spicy Bean Burgers

TURKEY CLUB SANDWICH

PREP TIME: 3 minutes
TOTAL TIME: 3 minutes
Makes 1 serving

Spread 2 tablespoons of hummus on 2 slices of rye bread. Layer 3 ounces turkey breast deli meat, 1 slice turkey bacon, 2 slices fresh avocado, sliced tomato, lettuce on top of 1 slice. Layer the remaining slice on top.

NUTRITION (*per serving*): 390 calories, 31 g Protein, 39 g carbohydrates, 5 g Fiber, 2 g sugar, 12 g fat, 2 g Saturated Fat, 745 mg sodium

PEPPERONI MUSHROOM PITA PIZZA

PREP TIME: 2 minutes
TOTAL TIME: 10 minutes
Makes 1 serving

Heat the oven or toaster oven to 400°F. Set 1 6-inch whole-wheat pita on a baking sheet, arrange 6 thin slices of tomato on top, and dot with 1½ oz. fresh mozzarella. Spread ⅓ cup mushrooms and 1½ ounces of turkey pepperoni all over and top with 6 small basil leaves. Bake until golden brown, 6 to 8 minutes. Remove from the oven, cut into 4 wedges, and serve immediately.

NUTRITION (*per serving*): 420 calories, 28 g protein, 42 g carbohydrates, 7 g fiber, 4 g sugar, 17 g fat, 8 g saturated fat, 1106 mg sodium

SEAFOOD SALAD

PREP TIME: 5 minutes
TOTAL TIME: 5
Makes 4 servings

- ½ cup mayonnaise
- 2 tablespoons chopped tarragon
- 1 tablespoon lime juice + wedges for serving
- 1 teaspoon country Dijon mustard
- ½ teaspoon ground turmeric
- ¼ teaspoon cayenne pepper
- ½ Granny Smith apple, finely chopped
- 1 rib celery, finely chopped
- 1 small shallot, finely chopped
- 1 pound cooked crab meat
- 1 cup baby arugula
- 4 whole grain pitas

In a medium bowl, whisk together the mayonnaise, tarragon, lime juice, mustard, turmeric, and cayenne. Fold in the apple, celery, shallot, and crab. Divide the arugula among the pita (in the pockets, if desired) and top with the crab salad. Serve with the chips.

NUTRITION (*per serving*): 478 calories, 30 g protein, 60 g carbs, 7 g fiber, 11 g sugar, 13 g fat, 2 g sat fat, 1297 mg sodium

SLOW COOKER VEGGIE CHILI

PREP TIME: 15 minutes
TOTAL TIME: 4 hours 15 minutes
Makes 8 servings

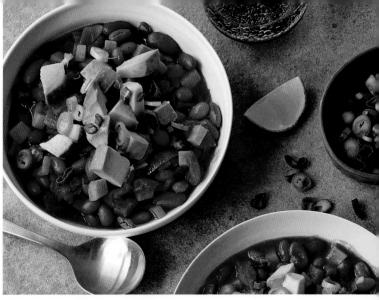

- 1 can (28 ounces) diced tomatoes
- 1 can (15 ounces) red kidney beans
- 1 can (15 ounces) pinto beans
- 1 can (15 ounces) chickpeas
- 1 can (15 ounces) white beans
- 2 small zucchini, chopped
- 2 bell peppers (any color), chopped
- 1 medium onion, chopped
- 1 large carrot, coarsely shredded
- 1 can (4 ounces) chopped green chilies
- 3 cloves garlic, minced
- 1 tablespoon chili powder
- 1 teaspoon ground cumin
- ½ teaspoon ground cayenne
- 8 ounces smoked tofu, diced
- 1 cup plain 2% Greek yogurt
- 1 cup shredded cheddar cheese
- 2 scallions, thinly sliced
- 2 slices fresh avocado

In a 6-quart slow cooker, stir together the tomatoes with juice, beans with liquid, zucchini, bell pepper, onion, carrot, green chilies, garlic, chili powder, cumin, and cayenne. Cover and cook until the vegetables are tender, 4 hours on high or 6 hours on low.

Divide the tofu among 8 bowls, ladle in the chili and top each with 2 tablespoons of the yogurt and cheese, and a sprinkling of scallions.

Top with avocado.

NUTRITION (*per serving*): 435 calories, 26 g protein, 58 g carbohydrates, 16 g fiber, 10 g sugar, 10 g fat, 4 g saturated fat, 798 mg sodium

PB&J PARFAIT

PREP TIME: 10 minutes
TOTAL TIME: 40
Makes: 2½ cups, 8 servings

- 2 cups rolled oats
- ¾ cup unsalted peanuts
- ⅓ cup flax seeds
- Pinch salt
- ¼ cup powdered peanut butter
- 3 tablespoons olive oil
- 2 tablespoons strawberry all-fruit spread (such as Polaner)
- 1 teaspoon vanilla
- ½ cup raisins
- 6 cups plain low fat Greek yogurt

Heat the oven to 250°F. In a large bowl, combine the oats, peanuts, flax seeds, and salt.

In a small saucepan over medium, combine the peanut butter, olive oil, fruit spread, and vanilla. Stir until combined and smooth. Pour over the dry ingredients and toss together. Spread in an even layer on a baking sheet and bake for 30 minutes, stirring every 10 minutes. Let cool to room temperature and stir in the raisins.

Serve ⅓ cup granola with cup yogurt.

NUTRITION (*per serving*): 399 calories, 24 g protein, 36 g carbohydrates, 5 g fiber, 16 g sugar, 19 g fat, 4 g saturated fat, 96 mg sodium

BLACK BEAN AND BROCCOLI BURRITO

PREP TIME: 10 minutes
TOTAL TIME: 60 minutes
Makes 6 servings

- 1 pound broccoli florets
- 2 tablespoons olive oil
- 1 yellow onion, sliced
- ½ to 1 Serrano chile, seeded and minced
- 1 clove garlic, sliced
- 2 cans (15 ounces each) low-sodium black beans, drained and rinsed
- 1 can (10 ounces) enchilada sauce, red or green
- ½ cup water
- 1 teaspoon ground cumin
- ½ teaspoon ground black pepper
- Kosher salt
- 1¼ cup cooked brown rice
- ¼ cup chopped cilantro leaves
- 6 (8") multigrain wraps
- 12 ounces smoked tofu, crumbled
- Hot sauce (optional)

Heat the oven to 425°F. Toss the broccoli with 1 tablespoon of the oil and roast until tender and browned, about 20 minutes. Remove from the oven and set aside.

In a large skillet, heat the remaining tablespoon oil over medium. Add the onion, chile, and garlic and cook until the onion begins to soften, about 5 minutes. Add the beans, enchilada sauce, water, cumin, black pepper, and pinch of salt and bring to a simmer. Reduce the heat and cook until the mixture thickens, about 25 minutes.

Stir the rice and cilantro together and divide among the wraps. Top with the bean mixture, broccoli, crumbled tofu, and hot sauce, if desired. Wrap the burritos up and serve.

NUTRITION (*per serving*): 512 calories, 25 g protein, 60 g carbohydrates, 15 g fiber, 4 g sugar, 16 g fat, 6.5 g saturated fat, 904 mg sodium

SLOW COOKER BBQ PULLED CHICKEN SALAD

PREP TIME: 5 minutes
TOTAL TIME: 4 hours 5 minutes
Makes 4 servings

- 1½ cups tomato puree or crushed tomatoes
- 1 large carrot, grated
- ¼ cup apple cider vinegar
- 2 tablespoons molasses
- 2 teaspoons smoked or sweet paprika
- 1 teaspoon Dijon mustard
- ½ teaspoon sea salt
- ½ teaspoon ground cayenne
- 1 small red onion, thinly sliced
- 1 pound boneless, skinless chicken breast
- 3 cups of salad greens
- 2 Tbs vinaigrette dressing
- ¼ cup diced avocado

In a slow cooker, combine the tomato sauce, carrot, vinegar, molasses, paprika, mustard, salt, and cayenne until smooth. Add the onion and nestle the chicken in the mixture, spooning a little over the top. Cover and cook on low until the chicken is very tender and reaches 165°F, about 4 hours on high. The chicken should be able to be pulled apart with a fork.

Remove the chicken from the sauce and set on a cutting board. Shred with two forks (or put into a bowl and shred with a handheld mixer) and return to the slow cooker. Mix until evenly coated with sauce.

Serve over dressed salad greens

NUTRITION (*per serving*): 394 calories, 28 g protein, 33 g carb, 9 g fiber, 16 g sugar, 17 g fat, 3 g saturated fat, 839 mg sodium

TIP: Pulled chicken freezes well, and this recipe easily doubles. Make a big batch and freeze half for a fast weeknight dinner.

EGG SALAD WRAPS

PREP TIME: 10 minutes
TOTAL TIME: 10 minutes
Makes 2 servings

- ⅓ cup plain low-fat Greek yogurt
- 2 tablespoons golden raisins
- 2 sliced scallions
- 2 teaspoons chia seeds
- 1 teaspoon Dijon mustard
- 1 teaspoon ground turmeric
- ½ teaspoon curry powder
- ¼ teaspoon kosher salt
- ¼ teaspoon ground black pepper
- 4 hard-boiled eggs, chopped
- 2 8-inch whole wheat tortillas
- 2 tablespoons cilantro leaves
- 2 teaspoons pumpkin seeds
- 2 Bibb or butter lettuce leaves

In a medium bowl, mix the yogurt, raisins, scallions, chia seeds, mustard, turmeric, curry powder, salt, and pepper. Stir in the eggs.

Set the tortillas on a work surface. Divide the egg mixture between them, spreading along the bottom third of the tortillas. Top each with the cilantro and pumpkin seeds, and set a lettuce leaf on top. Roll up from the bottom, tucking in the sides as you go.

NUTRITION (*per serving*): 404 calories, 23 g protein, 38 g carbs, 6 g fiber, 11 g sugar, 18 g fat, 5 g sat fat, 770 mg sodium

TUNA SALAD SANDWICH

PREP TIME: 3 minutes
TOTAL TIME: 3 minutes
Makes 1 serving

In a small bowl, combine ¾ cup water-packed canned tuna (drained) with ⅓ fresh avocado, mashed. Spread over two slices of whole grain bread.

NUTRITION (*per serving*): 389 calories, 37 g protein, 35 g carbohydrates, 8 g fiber, 6 g sugar, 13g fat, 3 g saturated fat, 617 mg sodium

SPICY BEAN BURGERS

PREP TIME: 10 minutes
TOTAL TIME: 1 hour 25 minutes
Makes 4 servings

- 1 small white onion, quartered
- 1 can (15.5 ounces) red kidney beans, drained and rinsed
- ½ cup whole-wheat panko breadcrumbs
- 3 scoops pea protein powder
- 1 teaspoon chili powder
- 1 teaspoon ground cumin
- ½ teaspoon cayenne pepper
- ½ teaspoon kosher salt
- ¼ teaspoon ground black pepper
- 1 egg, lightly beaten
- 1 tablespoon canola oil
- 4 whole wheat buns
- 1 avocado, sliced
- ½ cup sliced pimiento peppers or 2 roasted red pepper halves
- 4 lettuce leaves

Pulse the onion in a food processor until finely chopped, about 10 seconds. Add half the beans and process until they're a chunky puree, about 10 seconds. Transfer the mixture to a large bowl. Add the remaining beans, bread crumbs, protein powder, chili powder, cumin, cayenne, salt, and black pepper. Mix in the egg until well combined. With wet hands, form the mixture into 4 patties. Chill for 1 hour.

Heat the oil in a large nonstick skillet over medium-high. Add the patties and cook until browned, 5 to 7 minutes. Flip, and cook 4 to 6 minutes more.

Meanwhile, lightly toast the rolls. Transfer the cooked patties to the bottom rolls. Top each patty with ¼ of the avocado, ¼ of the pimientos, and 1 lettuce leaf. Close with the top roll.

NUTRITION (*per serving*): 474 calories, 24 g protein, 64 g carbohydrates, 17 g fiber, 15 g sugar, 15 g fat, 2 g saturated fat, 523 mg sodium

▶ DINNERS

69 Frank Steak with Edamame, Black Pepper, and Scallions

70 Chicken and Soup

72 Vegetable Omelet

70 Spaghetti and Meatballs

71 Greek Chicken and Vegetable Bake

71 Tofu Stir-Fry with Peanut Sauce

72 Italian Tilapia, Spinach and Tomato Packets

72 Steak Burrito Bowl

73 Crab Cake Meal

73 Baja Fish and Apple Salsa Tacos

74 Chipotle Chili Turkey Burgers

74 Broiled Pork Tenderloin with Cinnamon-Roasted Carrots

74 Turkey Wrap

FLANK STEAK WITH EDAMAME, BLACK PEPPER, AND SCALLIONS

PREP TIME: 10 minutes ❯ TOTAL TIME: 45 minutes ❯ Makes 4 servings

12 ounces flank steak

2 tablespoons rice wine vinegar

1 tablespoon sesame oil

1 tablespoon minced fresh ginger

2 teaspoons minced fresh garlic

3 cups fresh or thawed frozen edamame

¼ teaspoon salt

¼ teaspoon ground black pepper

2 scallions, thinly sliced

1 baked sweet potato

1 teaspoon unsalted butter

1. **Using a knife, pierce the beef all over. In a large bowl, combine the vinegar, oil, ginger, and garlic. Add the steak and marinate for 15 minutes at room temperature or up to 8 hours in the refrigerator, turning occasionally.**

2. **Position an oven rack 6 inches from the broiler element and heat the broiler to high. Line a large rimmed baking sheet with foil and mist with cooking spray.**

3. **Remove the steak from the marinade and place on the baking sheet. Broil until lightly charred around the edges, about 4 minutes. Flip, and broil until charred around the edges and cooked to your liking, about 4 minutes more for medium. Remove steak to a cutting board and rest 5 minutes before slicing.**

4. **Pour the marinade into a small skillet and bring to a simmer over medium heat. Cook until reduced by half, about 4 minutes. Add the edamame, salt, and pepper and cook until heated through, 2 minutes.**

5. **Thinly slice the steak against the grain and pour the edamame over the top. Sprinkle with the scallions. Serve with sweet potato topped with butter.**

NUTRITION (*per serving*): 463 calories, 32 g protein, 39 g carbohydrates, 9 g fiber, 9 g sugars, 19 g fat, 5 g saturated fat, 280 mg sodium

CHICKEN AND SOUP

PREP TIME: 15 minutes
TOTAL TIME: 15 minute
Makes 1 serving

Combine 1 cup Miso soup (commercially prepared) with 4 ounces rotisserie chicken. Serve with 1 small baked russet potato topped with 1 teaspoon of unsalted butter.

NUTRITION (*per serving*): 581 calories, 47 g protein, 45 g carbohydrates, 5 g fiber, 3 g sugar, 25 g fat, 7 g saturated fat, 1228 mg sodium

VEGETABLE OMELET

PREP TIME: 5 minutes
TOTAL TIME: 5 minutes
Makes 1 serving

In a small bowl, whisk together 3 large eggs. Stir in 1 cup cooked vegetables (onions, peppers, mushrooms) and a pinch of chili powder. In a large skillet over medium high heat, add the egg mixture. Cook for 5 minutes or until set. Serve with one slice of whole grain toast with 1 table-spoon natural peanut butter.

NUTRITION (*per serving*): 598 calories, 30 g protein, 39 g carbohydrates, 11 g fiber, 6g sugar, 34 g fat, 9 g saturated fat, 853 mg sodium

SPAGHETTI AND MEATBALLS

PREP TIME: 10 minutes
TOTAL TIME: 10 minutes
Makes 1 serving

Combine 1 cup cooked whole wheat pasta with ½ cup marinara sauce, 4 ounces cooked meatballs and 2 cups steamed broccoli.

NUTRITION (*per serving*): 581 calories, 30 g protein, 77 g carbohydrate, 16 g fiber, 22 g sugar, 22 g fat, 5 g saturated fat, 1228 mg sodium

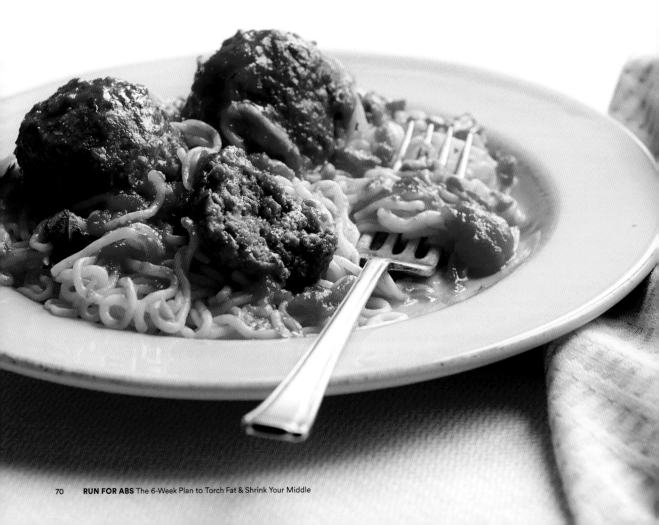

GREEK CHICKEN AND VEGETABLE BAKE

PREP TIME: 15 minutes
TOTAL TIME: 1 hour
Makes 4 servings

- 4 skinless, split, bone-in chicken breasts, trimmed (about 1½ pounds)
- 1 medium orange bell pepper, seeded and cut into 8 wedges
- 1 medium red bell pepper, seeded and cut into 8 wedges
- 1 medium yukon gold potato, cut into 8 wedges
- 1 medium red onion, cut into 8 wedges
- ⅔ cup pitted kalamata olives, coarsely chopped
- 1 lemon, peel grated then juiced
- 1 tablespoon extra virgin olive oil
- 1 tablespoon minced garlic
- 1 tablespoon chopped fresh oregano
- ¾ teaspoon paprika
- ½ teaspoon freshly ground black pepper
- ½ cup prepared quinoa

1. Preheat the oven to 400°F. Line a large rimmed baking sheet with foil.

2. Place the chicken on one side of the baking sheet and the bell peppers, potato, onion, and olives on the other. In a bowl, whisk together the lemon zest and juice, oil, garlic, oregano, paprika and pepper. Drizzle over the chicken and vegetables, and toss to coat.

3. Roast, turning the chicken and stirring the vegetables halfway through cooking, until a meat thermometer registers 165°F when inserted into the thickest part of the chicken (not touching bone), about 45 minutes.

4. Arrange a chicken breast and a quarter of the vegetables on each of 4 plates. Serve with quinoa.

NUTRITION (*per serving*): 480 calories, 32 g protein, 40 g carbohydrates, 6 g fiber, 5 g sugars, 23 g fat, 3 g saturated fat, 1016 mg sodium

TOFU STIR-FRY WITH PEANUT SAUCE

PREP TIME: 10 minutes
TOTAL TIME: 25 minutes
Makes 2 serving

- 6 ounces firm tofu, cubed
- 1½ cups sugar snap peas
- 1 cup asparagus sliced on the diagonal
- ½ cup sliced mushrooms
- 2 teaspoons grated fresh ginger
- 2 clove garlic, minced
- ¼ cup reduced sodium soy sauce
- 2 tablespoons creamy peanut butter
- 2 tablespoons white wine vinegar
- 2 teaspoons brown sugar
- ½ teaspoon ground cayenne
- 1 cup cooked whole-grain spaghetti
- 1 cup julienned (matchsticks) carrots
- 2 cups baby spinach, washed and dried
- ¼ cup tomato, diced
- ½ cup cucumber, sliced
- 1 tablespoon vinaigrette

In a large nonstick skillet coated with cooking spray, cook the tofu over medium heat, stirring frequently, until browned, about 5 minutes. Remove from the pan and set aside. Spray the pan again with cooking spray and add the peas, asparagus, mushrooms, ginger, and garlic and cook, stirring frequently, until crisp-tender, about 5 minutes.

In a small bowl, combine ¼ cup of water with the soy sauce, peanut butter, vinegar, sugar, and cayenne, stirring to combine. Pour the sauce over the vegetables and simmer for 1 minute. Add back the tofu, and stir in the pasta and carrots to coat and heat through, about 1 minute.

For side salad, toss together 2 cups baby spinach with ¼ cup tomato, ½ cup sliced cucumber and dress with vinaigrette.

NUTRITION (*per serving*): 443 calories, 27 g protein, 54 g carbohydrates, 14 g fiber, 14 g sugars, 18 g fat, 3 g saturated fat, 515 mg sodium

ITALIAN TILAPIA, SPINACH AND TOMATO PACKETS

PREP TIME: 5 minutes
TOTAL TIME: 25 minutes
Makes 6 servings

- 12 ounces baby spinach leaves (12 cups)
- 6 tilapia fillets (about 2 ½ pounds)
- 1½ teaspoons kosher salt
- 6 cloves garlic, thinly sliced
- 1 can (14 ounces) diced tomatoes with basil
- 1½ teaspoons Italian seasoning
- 6 tablespoons extra-virgin olive oil
- 3 cups cooked brown rice

1. Position 2 oven racks in the upper and lower thirds of the oven. Preheat the oven to 400°F.

2. Tear six 12 × 18-inch pieces of aluminum foil and mist with cooking spray. Fold a sheet in half and open like a book. Mound 2 cups spinach in the center of one half. Top with the tilapia, sprinkle with ¼ teaspoon salt and top with 1 of the sliced cloves of garlic. Spoon ¼ cup tomatoes over the fish and sprinkle with ¼ teaspoon Italian seasoning. Drizzle with 1 tablespoon of the oil and fold the empty half of the foil over the fish. Fold over the edges tightly on all three sides to retain the steam. Transfer to a large rimmed baking sheet. Repeat with the remaining aluminum foil and ingredients, placing 3 packets per baking sheet.

3. Bake the packets until they puff up, about 10 minutes. Remove one packet and open carefully, there will be steam. Check that the fish is fully cooked through and opaque and the spinach is wilted. If more time is needed, reseal the packet and place back in the oven for a couple minutes more.

4. Serve each person a packet and let them open it at the table. Serve with ½ cup brown rice each.

NUTRITION (*per serving*): 454 calories, 42 g protein, 33 g carbohydrates, 4 g fiber, 2 g sugars, 18 g fat, 3 g saturated fat, 898 mg sodium

STEAK BURRITO BOWL

PREP TIME: 10 minutes
TOTAL TIME: 25 minutes
Makes 4 servings

- 1 teaspoon olive oil
- 1 teaspoon chipotle seasoning
- ½ teaspoon black pepper
- 12 ounces lean flank steak, trimmed
- 4 cups cooked brown rice
- 1 can (15 ounces) black beans, rinsed and drained
- 2 cups shredded romaine lettuce
- ½ cup salsa
- 1 avocado, diced
- ¾ cup shredded Cheddar or Cheddar-Jack

Prepare a grill for medium-high heat cooking. Brush and oil the grates. In a small bowl, combine the oil, chipotle seasoning, and black pepper. Rub all over the steak and grill, turning once, until a thermometer inserted in the center registers 145°F for medium-rare, about 10 minutes. Transfer the steak to a cutting board and let sit 5 minutes before slicing into thin strips against the grain.

Evenly divide the rice among 4 bowls. Top with the steak, beans, lettuce, salsa, avocado, and cheese.

NUTRITION (*per serving*): 508 calories, 29 g protein, 62 g carbohydrates, 9 g fiber, 2 g sugars, 16 g fat, 5 g saturated fat, 441 mg sodium

CRAB CAKE MEAL

PREP TIME: 15 minutes
TOTAL TIME: 60 minutes
Makes 2 servings

- 1 sweet potato, cut into ½-inch-thick wedges
- 1½ tablespoons olive oil, divided
- ¼ teaspoon cayenne pepper
- 1 egg
- ¼ cup whole wheat bread panko crumbs
- 1 tablespoon mayonnaise
- 1 teaspoon Dijon mustard
- ½ teaspoon crab-boil seasoning
- 8 ounces lump crab meat
- 1 scallion, greens only, chopped
- 2 teaspoons white wine vinegar
- 1 tablespoon chopped fresh parsley or cilantro
- ½ teaspoon ground turmeric
  Kosher salt and ground black pepper
- 1 medium yellow squash, cut into ribbons with a vegetable peeler
- 1 can (15 ounces) no-salt-added chickpeas, rinsed and drained

Heat the oven to 450°F. Toss the sweet potato with 1½ teaspoons of the olive oil and cayenne. Spread on a baking sheet and roast until golden and tender, about 35 minutes.

In a medium bowl, stir together the egg, 1 tablespoon of the mayonnaise, mustard, and seasoning. Stir in the crab meat and scallion greens and form into 4 small patties.

Heat a large skillet over medium and spray with cooking spray. Cook the crab cakes until golden, about 5 minutes per side.

In a medium bowl, stir together the olive oil, vinegar, parsley, and a pinch of salt and pepper. Toss the squash ribbons and chickpeas in this mixture and set aside.

Serve the crab cakes alongside the squash salad and sweet potato wedges.

NUTRITION (*per serving*): 559 calories, 41 g protein, 50 g carbohydrates, 10 g fiber, 7 g sugars, 21 g total fat, 3 g saturated fat, 883 mg sodium

BAJA FISH AND APPLE SALSA TACOS

PREP TIME: 10 minutes
TOTAL TIME: 25 minutes
Makes 4 servings

- 2 tablespoons olive oil; more for grill
- ½ teaspoon chili powder
- 1½ pound cod fillets (or similar white flaky fish), cut into 4 pieces
- 1 large sweet crisp apple, such as Honeycrisp, quartered and cored
- 2 cobs fresh corn, shucked
- ½ medium red onion, thickly sliced
- 1 small jicama, peeled and diced (about 1 cup)
- 3 Tbsp fresh lime juice
- 1 Tbsp chopped cilantro leaves
  Salt and pepper to taste
- 8 whole wheat tortillas (7-inch)

Prepare a grill or grill pan over medium heat. Brush and oil the grates. Stir together the oil and chili powder. Coat the fish with this mixture, season with salt and pepper and set aside.

Grill the apple, corn, and onion until charred and tender, about 7 minutes. When cool enough to handle, dice the apple, cut the corn kernels from the cob, and chop the onion and transfer to a medium bowl. Stir in the jicama, lime juice, and cilantro; season with salt and pepper. Set aside to let the flavors meld.

Grill the fish until opaque, about 4 minutes per side. Divide the fish between the tortillas, top with the apple salsa, and serve.

NUTRITION (*per serving*): 551 calories, 41 g protein, 65 g carbohydrates, 10 g fiber, 9 g sugar, 15 g fat, 3 g saturated fat, 800 mg sodium

CHIPOTLE CHILI TURKEY BURGERS

PREP TIME: 5 minutes
TOTAL TIME: 15 minutes
Makes 4 servings

- 1 pound ground turkey (not ground turkey breast)
- 3 canned chipotle chili peppers in adobo sauce, chopped
- ½ cup finely chopped white onion (about ½ medium onion)
- 2 cloves garlic, minced
- ½ teaspoon kosher salt
  Canola oil, for the grill
- 4 large hearty, whole-grain buns, sliced
- 1 avocado, sliced

Prepare a grill for medium-high heat. In a large bowl, add the turkey, peppers, onion, garlic, and salt and mix until thoroughly combined. Using wet hands, form the mixture into 4 patties.

Brush the grill grates with the oil. Cook the patties on the grill, with the lid closed, until good grill marks form, 5 minutes. Flip and top each patty with 2 Tbsp. queso fresco. Close the lid and cook until the burgers reach an internal temperature of 165°F, about 5 minutes more.

Meanwhile, lightly toast the buns. Transfer the patties to the bottom buns and top each with the avocado slices and close with the top bun.

NUTRITION (*per serving*): 396 calories, 28 g protein, 28 g carbohydrates, 6 g fiber, 5 g sugar, 21 g fat, 4 g saturated fat, 698 mg sodium

BROILED PORK TENDERLOIN WITH CINNAMON-ROASTED CARROTS

PREP TIME: 5 minutes
TOTAL TIME: 35 minutes
Makes 4 servings

- 1 tablespoon olive oil
- ½ teaspoon ground cinnamon
- ¼ teaspoon coarse salt
- 1 pound baby carrots
- 5 ounces pork tenderloin
- 1 slice 100% whole grain bread
- ½ of a medium avocado, sliced
- ½ cup cottage cheese

1. **Preheat the oven to 425°F. Arrange the carrots on a large rimmed baking sheet. Drizzle with the oil and sprinkle with the cinnamon and salt. Toss to coat.**

2. **Roast the carrots, stirring occasionally, until tender and lightly browned, about 30 minutes.**

3. **During the last 15 minutes of roasting, add the pork tenderloin.**

4. **Meanwhile toast the bread, then spread it with the cottage cheese and sliced avocado.**

Nutrition (per serving) 521 calories, 49 g protein, 38 g carbohydrates, 7 g fiber, 13 g sugars, 21 g fat, 1.5 g saturated fat, 697 mg sodium

TURKEY WRAP

PREP TIME: 7 minutes
TOTAL TIME: 7 minutes
Makes 1 serving

On one large whole grain tortilla (12-inch) layer 4 ounces sliced turkey breast, 1 tablespoon feta cheese, ¼ cup baby spinach, 1 tablespoon sliced olives, ¼ cup diced tomatoes, 1 tablespoon vinaigrette dressing. Fold up both sides of the tortilla and roll. Serve with one medium apple and 1 tablespoon natural almond butter.

NUTRITION (*per serving*): 575 calories, 36 g protein, 54 g carbohydrates, 11 g fiber, 27 g sugar, 31 g fat, 7 g saturated fat, 1289 mg sodium

▶ SNACKS

75 Recovery Smoothie

75 Homemade Energy Bites

75 Chocolate Ricotta
   Mousse Dip with Fruit

75 Beefed Up Trail Mix

76 Cherry Berry-Almond Smoothie

77 Sweet 'N' Spicy Tropical Smoothie

77 Crispy Roasted Spiced
   Chickpeas with String Cheese

75 Cottage Cheese Parfait

77 Egg and Hummus

77 Date Balls

RECOVERY SMOOTHIE

PREP TIME: 5 minutes
TOTAL TIME: 5 minutes
Makes 2 servings

In a blender, combine ½ cup brewed and chilled coffee, 1 cup full-fat plain Greek yogurt, 1 small banana, ½ avocado, 1 scoop chocolate protein powder, ½ teaspoon fresh ginger, and ½ cup ice. Blend until smooth.

NUTRITION (*per serving*): 263 calories, 23 g protein, 21 g carbohydrates, 4 g fiber, 12 g sugars, 11 g total fat, 4 g saturated fat, 76 mg sodium

HOMEMADE ENERGY BITES

PREP TIME: 10 minutes
TOTAL TIME: 15 minutes
Makes 8 servings

In a food processor, add 1½ cups pitted dates, 3 scoops protein powder, ¼ cup unsweetened cocoa powder, ¼ cup nut butter, ½ teaspoon cinnamon, zest of 1 medium orange, and a pinch of salt and pulse until combined. Form into ¾-inch balls and roll in ¼ cup unsweetened shredded coconut. Makes about 24 balls.

NUTRITION (*per serving*): 207 calories, 12 g protein, 29 g carbohydrates, 5 g fiber, 22 g sugar, 7 g fat, 2.5 g saturated fat, 56 mg sodium

CHOCOLATE RICOTTA MOUSSE DIP WITH FRUIT

PREP TIME: 5 minutes
TOTAL TIME: 5 minutes
Makes 1 serving

In a small bowl, combine ½ cup part skim ricotta cheese, 1 tablespoon unsweetened cocoa powder, 1 teaspoon maple syrup, and ¼ teaspoon ground cinnamon and stir until completely combined. Serve with 1 cup strawberries, pineapple, or bananas.

NUTRITION (*per serving*): 248 calories, 16 g protein, 26 g carbohydrates, 5 g fiber, 12 g sugar, 11 g fat, 7 g saturated fat, 158 mg sodium

BEEFED UP TRAIL MIX

PREP TIME: 10 minutes
TOTAL TIME: 25 minutes
Makes 12 servings

In a large bowl, toss together 6 cups air popped popcorn, 4 ounces beef jerky (coarsely chopped), ¾ cup toasted pecans (coarsely chopped), 4 ounces natural fruit leather (coarsely chopped), ⅓ cup roasted salted pumpkin seeds (pepitas) until well combined.

NUTRITION (*per serving*): 154 calories, 5 g protein, 13 g carbohydrates, 2 g fiber, 7 g sugar, 9 g fat, 2 g saturated fat, 243 mg sodium

CHERRY BERRY-ALMOND SMOOTHIE

PREP TIME: 5 minutes ❯ **TOTAL TIME: 5 minutes** ❯ **Makes 1 serving**

½ cup frozen tart cherries	1 tablespoon natural almond butter
3 tablespoons 2% Greek yogurt	½ teaspoon pure vanilla extract
¼ cup pomegranate-cherry 100% juice	¼ teaspoon ground cinnamon
¼ cup fresh or frozen blueberries	¼ teaspoon ground turmeric

In a blender, combine all the ingredients and blend until smooth. Divide between 2 glasses.

NUTRITION (*per serving*): 250 calories, 12 g protein, 28 g carbohydrates, 4 g fiber, 22 g sugars, 11 g fat, 2 g saturated fat, 50 mg sodium

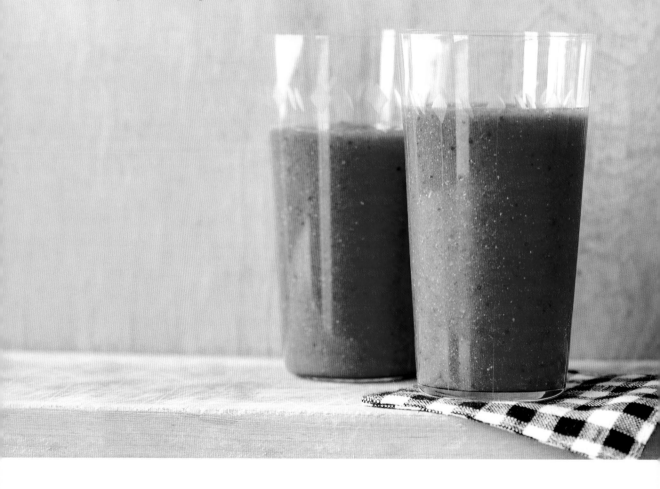

SWEET 'N' SPICY TROPICAL SMOOTHIE

RECIPE BY KHALIL HYMORE QUASHA

PREP TIME: 5 minutes
TOTAL TIME: 5 minutes
Makes 1 serving

- ½ cup frozen pineapple and/or mango
- ½ ripe avocado
- ¼ cup coconut water
- ½ scoop whey protein powder
- 1 tablespoon lemon juice
- 1-inch piece fresh ginger
- ⅛ teaspoon ground cayenne

In a blender combine all the ingredients and blend until smooth. Divide between 2 glasses.

NUTRITION (*per serving*): 199 calories, 10 g protein, 24 g carbohydrates, 6 g fiber, 14 g sugars, 8 g fat, 2 g saturated fat, 87 mg sodium

CRISPY ROASTED SPICED CHICKPEAS WITH STRING CHEESE

PREP TIME: 5 minutes
TOTAL TIME: 35 minutes
Makes 2 servings

Heat the oven to 450°F. Spread 1 can (15 ounces) drained and rinsed chickpeas on paper towels and pat dry. Toss on a large rimmed baking sheet with 1 tablespoon olive oil, ½ teaspoon paprika, ¼ teaspoon each salt, pepper, and cumin to coat. Roast until browned and crisp, about 30 minutes. Let cool to crisp. Serve along with a stick of string cheese.

NUTRITION (*per serving*): 233 calories, 12 g protein, 20 g carbohydrates, 5 g fiber, 2 g sugars, 13 g total fat, 3 g saturated fat, 798 mg sodium

COTTAGE CHEESE PARFAIT

PREP TIME: 2 minutes
TOTAL TIME: 2 minutes
Makes 1 serving

In a tall glass, layer ½ cup cottage cheese, ¾ cup blueberries, and 1 tablespoon chopped walnuts.

NUTRITION (*per serving*): 177 calories, 16 g protein, 21 g carbohydrates, 4 g fiber, 15 g sugar, 6 g fat, 2 g saturated fat, 361 mg sodium

EGG AND HUMMUS

PREP TIME: 2 minutes
TOTAL TIME: 2 minutes
Makes 1 serving

One hard boiled egg with 2 tablespoons hummus and 5 whole grain crackers.

NUTRITION (*per serving*): 198 calories, 9 g protein, 14 g carbohydrates, 4 g fiber, 2 g sugar, 11 g fat, 3 g saturated fat, 309 mg sodium

DATE BALLS

PREP TIME: 15 minutes
TOTAL TIME: 20 minutes
Makes 6 servings

- ⅓ cup chopped dates
- 2 tablespoons sunflower seeds
- 2 tablespoons chopped macadamia nuts
- 2 tablespoons chopped cashews
- 2 tablespoons maple syrup
- 1 scoop vanilla or chocolate protein powder
- 1 tablespoon cacao nibs
- 1 teaspoon melted coconut oil
- 1 teaspoon unsweetened cocoa powder
- ½ teaspoon vanilla extract
- ¼ cup unsweetened shredded coconut

1. In a food processor, combine the dates, sunflower seeds, macadamia nuts, cashews, maple syrup, protein powder, cacao nibs, coconut oil, cocoa powder, and vanilla. Pulse for 30 seconds, stop to scrape down the sides of the bowl. Process until the ingredients form a ball about 30 seconds more.

2. Using your hands, roll the mixture into 12 balls, about 1 tablespoon each. Roll the balls in the coconut. Serve immediately, or store in an airtight container for up to 1 week.

NUTRITION (*per serving*): 154 calories, 6 g protein, 13 g carbohydrates, 2 g fiber, 10 g sugars, 9 g fat, 4 g saturated fat, 11 mg sodium

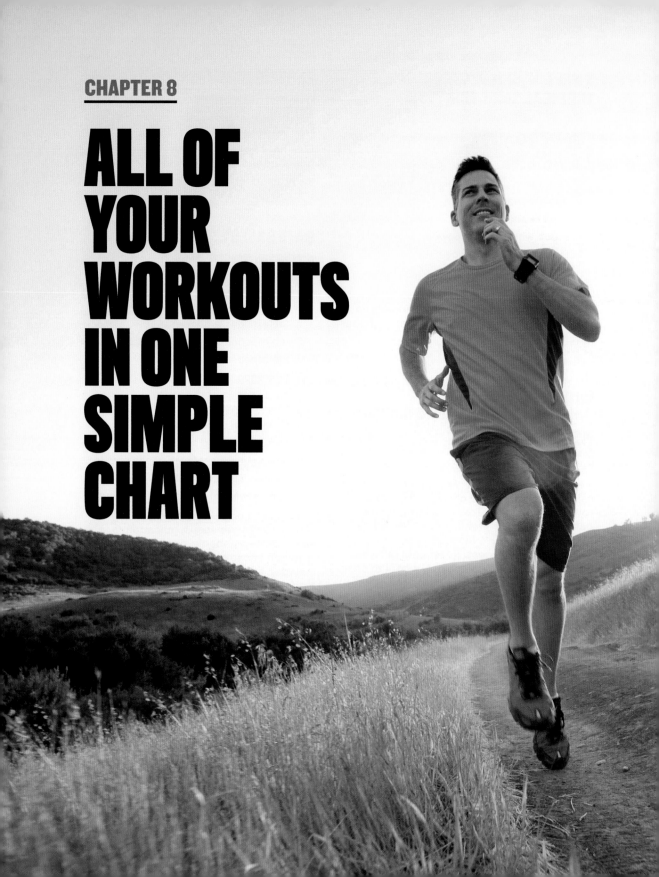

CHAPTER 8

ALL OF YOUR WORKOUTS IN ONE SIMPLE CHART

Day 1	Day 2	Day 3	Day 4	Day 5	Day 6	Day 7
Strength 2 Circuits Fast Run 1-3 miles	Off	Intervals 30s Hard 90s Recovery 5-6 Rounds	Strength 2 Circuits Fast Run 1-3 miles	Off	Hills 30s Uphill 90s Recovery 4-5 Rounds	Off

Day 8	Day 9	Day 10	Day 11	Day 12	Day 13	Day 14
Strength 2 Circuits Fast Run 1-3 miles	Off	Intervals 30s Hard 90s Recovery 6-7 Rounds	Strength 2 Circuits Fast Run 1-3 miles	Off	Hills 30s Uphill 90s Recovery 6-7 Rounds	Off

Day 15	Day 16	Day 17	Day 18	Day 19	Day 20	Day 21
Strength 2 Circuits Fast Run 1-3 miles	Off	Intervals 30s Hard 90s Recovery 7-8 Rounds	Strength 2 Circuits Fast Run 1-3 miles	Off	Hills 30s Uphill 90s Recovery 7-8 Rounds	Off

Day 22	Day 23	Day 24	Day 25	Day 26	Day 27	Day 28
Strength 3 Circuits Fast Run 1-3 miles	Off	Intervals 30s Hard 30s Recovery 3 Repeats, followed by 90s recovery 4-5 Rounds	Strength 3 Circuits Fast Run 1-3 miles	Off	Hills 30s Uphill 90s Recovery 8-9 Rounds	Off

Day 29	Day 30	Day 31	Day 32	Day 33	Day 34	Day 35
Strength 3 Circuits Fast Run 1-3 miles	Off	Intervals 30s Hard 30s Recovery 3 Repeats, followed by 90s recovery 5-6 Rounds	Strength 3 Circuits Fast Run 1-3 miles	Off	Hills 30s Uphill 90s Recovery 9-10 Rounds	Off

Day 36	Day 37	Day 38	Day 39	Day 40	Day 41	Day 42
Strength 3 Circuits Fast Run 1-3 miles	Off	Intervals 30s Hard 30s Recovery 3 Repeats, followed by 90s recovery 6-7 Rounds	Strength 3 Circuits Fast Run 1-3 miles	Off	Hills 30s Uphill 90s Recovery 10 Rounds	Off

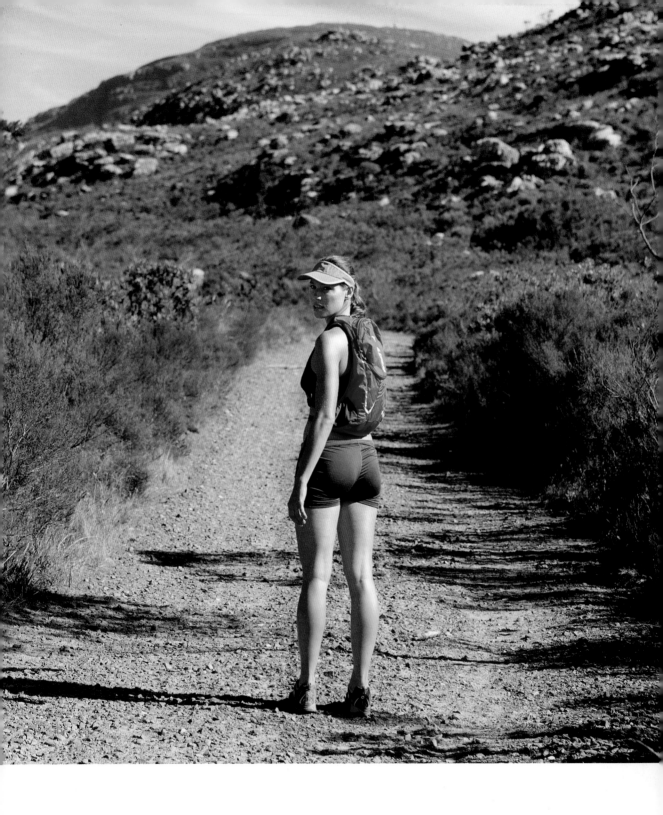